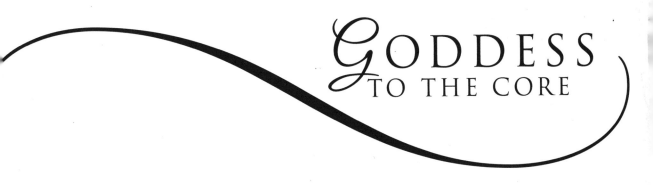

Many people have asked me how I founded Boot Camp for Goddesses.® My journey began on Christmas Eve in 1995 with a near-death experience. I suffered a rare ectopic pregnancy that was misdiagnosed, causing my uterus to rupture after being months into my pregnancy, which caused me to almost bleed to death. The doctors didn't expect me to survive. Technically, I died on the operating table. Although modern medicine saved my life, my dance with death changed me forever. Modern medicine could not heal the emotional wounds and the psychological scars, nor could it begin to answer all of my questions.

My conversations with God during my near-death experience led me into alignment with all human aspects of myself—spiritual, mental, emotional, and physical, and in that order. God asked me four questions: Spiritually, where did I disconnect from the source of God's love? Mentally, what were the belief systems that took me further away from God's love? Emotionally, when did I stop feeling worthy of God's love? And physically, why did I continually punish myself by not accepting God's love?

In my search for answers, I saw many doctors, specialists, therapists, and healers, and I spent thousands of dollars. Although all of these things helped me temporarily, they did not heal the core of my issues. I felt as if I were spinning my wheels, and I came to believe that the healing process should not take so long. My answers were found through working with indigenous people, listening to my own innate wisdom, and coming into alignment with God, Earth, and Christ consciousness, the sources that feed me love. Spirit guided me to share what I had experienced with other women.

The loss of my unborn child and the damage to my feminine organs, resulting in an inability to bear children, helped me to redefine fitness, beauty, and power for a healthy woman in the world today. I started rebuilding my personal connection to the physical and spiritual world. Spirit led me to spend more time with Mother Earth, the most powerful feminine healing source and goddess of all. I soon realized it wasn't necessary to travel the world or spend thousands of dollars on modern medicine.

The answers were right outside my door, in nature.

In searching for the answers to God's questions, I was able to heal myself. Then I noticed many women were having the same frustrating experience with our current system of healing. Most women were like mice on a wheel, working very hard but getting nowhere. They began to ask me for my secrets: how I had healed and integrated my past hurts, abuses, losses, and my near-death experience to become so whole, holy, and healthy.

I designed Boot Camp for Goddesses® as a result of my own healing. I soon realized the most successful approach was an intense week-long camp where women would immerse themselves in the healing process by answering the same four questions for themselves in a loving, supportive atmosphere without the distractions of daily life and circumstances that pull them back into the very situations they are trying to heal.

Many women assume that a boot camp is a place where I will beat them up and break them down, something they have come to believe they deserve. The tenderness and grace given them at Boot Camp for Goddesses® surprises most women. There, I help women to heal from the inside out. It is one of my core beliefs that we have all the answers within us, and my job is to empower women—to pull forth the power, beauty, mystery, and magic that lies within.

As a result of my fiery, energetic personality and my athletic background, I brought something new and different to the yoga and healing communities. Most of my life, I had been in touch with my Warrior side, yet I had denied certain aspects of myself—my true power: my feminine essence. When asked which side they are more likely to identify with, 70 out of 100 women say they are more in touch with their Warrior rather than their Goddess side. As women, if we are unable to be in touch or in tune with our feminine self, how can we even begin to be comfortable in our own bodies? How can we be fully empowered if we are not balanced? Women have become so disconnected from their core of being, from their feminine essence. With a true balance of Goddess and Warrior, I am able to bring women to new levels, both physically and emotionally, leading them to embrace and redefine the power of their femininity. While always holding on to the receptive energy of the feminine essence, I remain peaceful yet fierce, graceful yet powerful.

As low as painful life experiences can take us, they have the power to take us just as high. If we surrender and give up what is no longer of service to us, we allow ourselves to receive love—not just as an emotion but as the most powerful force and source—leading us to the expression of our true authentic self.

Sierra Bender

Praise for Sierra Bender and her
Boot Camp for Goddesses® *workshops*

Sierra's unique integrative program offers women a blend of ancient and modern, spiritual and physical tools for strengthening themselves from the inside out. When women leave her workshop at Omega, their transformation is absolutely visible!
> —Carla Goldstein, director of the Women's Leadership Center at the Omega Institute

Sierra Bender can only be described as a force of nature, an inspired teacher who has through direct experience created an astonishing technique of transformation certain to reveal the goddess within.
> —Wade Davis, explorer-in-residence, National Geographic Society
> and bestselling author of *One River* and *The Serpent and the Rainbow*

Sierra has seemingly interminable knowledge about how to help women "be women." She herself is challenging, compassionate, and radiantly confident, a model of how to balance the Warrior and Goddess energies women have.
> —Sharon M., Ph.D., Harvard Medical School executive coach for women

Sierra Bender is not an academic who was dying to teach because she was afraid of living; she is a "Warrior of Life" who can teach because she allowed nearly dying to release her to discover living.
> —Warren Farrell, Ph.D., author of *Why Men Are the Way They Are* and
> *Women Can't Hear What Men Don't Say*

The boot camp is all about what's right with you, not what's wrong with you. Quite simply, it was an oasis of calm and restoration in an otherwise crazy and draining world.
> —Beverly K., contributor for *People* magazine

Boot camp took us to the edge mentally, physically, and spiritually. We not only survived—by banding together, we kicked butt. Sharing difficult memories helped us heal and drew us closer as the week went on. These goddesses rule.
> —Judy D.

I had an amazing experience. I've already told my girlfriends that they must do this. And already Boot Camp for Goddesses is helping my marriage more than all the self-help books and couples' workshops we have done! So, thank you. What you have created is truly unique and special and so rich with gifts.

—Debbie B.

I met a new guy, and he actually called me a goddess … without me telling him anything about that part of my life. I thought it was pretty cool and that it was proof that I am carrying myself with the principles Sierra taught me—the essence of what it means to be a woman.

—Linda

Something has shifted at a deep level. I thought I was done with all the crying some time ago for this life, but these new tears are a new kind—mostly tears of relief and often joy. There is so much more to heal, let go, and draw forth. I can't even begin to thank you enough for your brilliance and courage. You have helped me begin to take back what is mine that was hidden or taken from me long ago.

—Marie D.

Sierra helped me to regain my power and learn to stand in my truth. Her energy is indescribable, but I'll try. It's kind of like eating chocolate while shopping and having an orgasm all at the same time! She is the most extraordinary woman I have ever met. I am finally on the journey I have been meant to take all my life.

—Tonya L.

The boot camp was all that I expected and so much more. Upon my arrival home, I was greeted by my boyfriend with so much love and respect, and he noticed this overall clarity about me. I applaud you, as you are a very beautiful, compassionate, and brave woman. You seem to have overcome some huge hurdles, and like the rest of us, you are continually learning and yearning to better your life.

—Shelley M.

It is so simple and yet extremely difficult to accept: the answer is not anywhere else but inside me. Women are blessed with the gift of intuition, and somehow we suppress it. Sierra guided me and the rest of the seekers to reconnect with this gift, this special power handed down to us by all goddesses. Today I am grounded in my own powerful feminine force full of love.

—Angelica S.

The 4 Body Fit concept that Sierra teaches is a powerful tool for healing, and I am grateful to be teaching this today. As Sierra says, "The issues are in the tissues."

—Mary C., RN ACE RYT

It was magical … All of my senses were awakened, and I felt connected to myself, nature, my family, and my job. I have been told by others that I am more compassionate and that I possess and radiate positive energy. These feelings and a sense of commitment are still with me today. I will always be grateful to Sierra for letting me "know my truth, see my truth, speak my truth, and feel my truth." I still begin every day with this mantra.

—Lori W.

My sister, daughter, and I attended Boot Camp for Goddesses together. One thing we all agreed on: some of it was work, but some of it, like dancing in the rain, was so much fun! Not only did we learn how to take care of ourselves as individuals but also as family members, and how to set boundaries, respect each other's time and space while still being kind and caring.

—Eve D.

You and your Boot Camp for Goddesses have touched my life in so many ways. It has truly been one of the most incredible experiences and it continues to be a very important part of me. I am a better person in all aspects of my life—wife, mother, daughter, friend, business partner, stranger. Your boot camp is about a way of life. It is now my life. Thank you!

—Linda

After Boot Camp for Goddesses, I felt more empowered, less bewildered, with more clarity and drive. Boot Camp for Goddesses was a gift to myself that I want to give to every woman I know. So, through example, I share my lessons: let go of what no longer serves you, and embrace the goddess within.

—Lori F.

I learned so much more than I expected. It was so affirming to know that what I thought was correct—I didn't need therapy or Xanax. I simply needed a way to replenish myself. And you showed me how to do that.

—Mary P.

Relationship / Home / Job

If we know what power is → we wouldn't give it away

Lead by example

Diva - express goal through art

What am I doing?

Why?

How is it effecting me?

GODDESS
TO THE CORE

An Inspired Workout to Maximize
Your Fitness, Beauty & Power

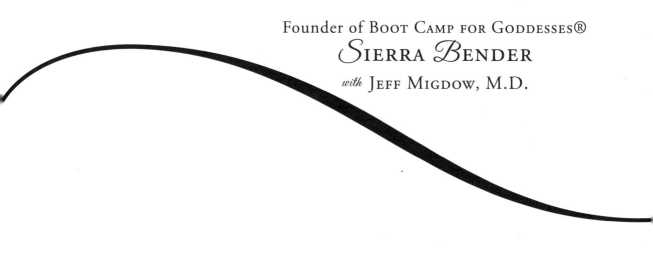

Founder of BOOT CAMP FOR GODDESSES®
SIERRA BENDER
with JEFF MIGDOW, M.D.

LLEWELLYN PUBLICATIONS ♣ WOODBURY, MINNESOTA

First Printing, 2009

FIRST EDITION

Book design by Rebecca Zins
Cover design by Lisa Novak
Cover photos by Felipe Riquelme
Illustrations by Llewellyn Art Department
Interior photos by Felipe Riquelme and Wendy McCrane Strang

The author gratefully acknowledges Kate Hanley for her inspiration and contribution.

Library of Congress Cataloging-in-Publication Data
Bender, Sierra.
 Goddess to the core : an inspired workout to maximize your fitness, beauty, and power / Sierra Bender ; with Jeff Migdow.
  p. cm.
 Includes bibliographical references and index.
 ISBN 978-0-7387-1503-2
 1. Physical fitness. 2. Self-care, Health. 3. Breathing exercises—Therapeutic use. 4. Spiritual exercises. I. Migdow, Jeffrey A.. II. Title.
 RA781.B412 2009
 613.7—dc22

2009043238

Llewellyn Publications
A Division of Llewellyn Worldwide, Ltd.
2143 Wooddale Drive, Dept. 978-0-7387-1503-2
Woodbury, MN 55125-2989
www.llewellyn.com

Printed in the United States of America

CONTENTS

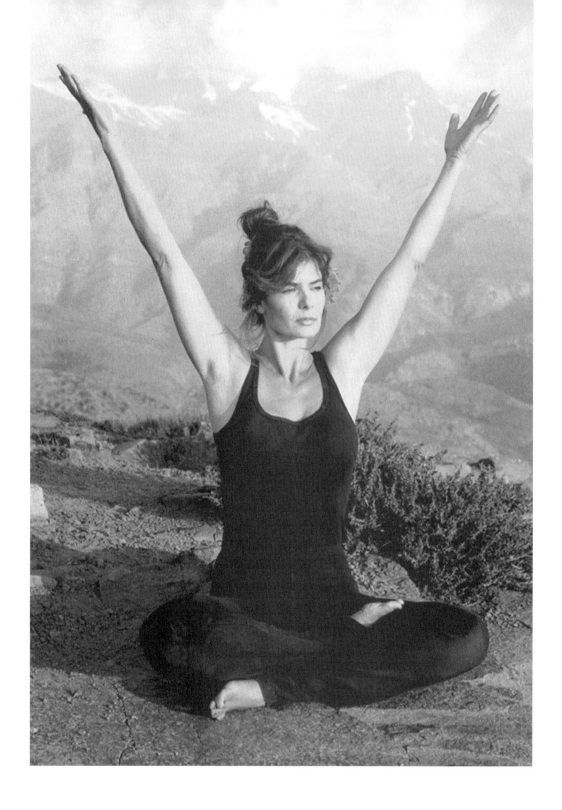

FOREWORD

One of our biggest problems with modern healing is that it only treats one body at a time. The medical doctor specializes in the physical body, and often in only one part of the body. Psychiatrists and psychologists treat only the mental and emotional bodies. Priests and rabbis work only on the spiritual body. In ancient times, healers worked with all dimensions of our lives with a wide array of tools:

- Prayer, fasting, ceremony, dancing, and vision quests to open up a dialog with Spirit.

- Meditation, mantra, and mindfulness to train the mental body.

- Breathing exercises, singing, chanting, dancing, drumming, and ceremony to work with the emotions.

- Movement, herbs, massage, body work, and nutrition to heal the physical body.

The root of this separation is that we have lost the feminine essence of Spirit in our society, religion, and healing. In ancient times, the healers and leaders of healing ceremonies were often medicine women, female shamans, oracles, and priestesses. But this female presence began to shift about 2,200 years ago as the patriarchal paradigm began to take over.

Fortunately, today we are experiencing a resurgence of feminine energy in healing, as seen in the rise in popularity of modalities such as acupuncture, homeopathy, Reiki, qigong, yoga, Ayurveda, herbal medicine, and homeopathy. These approaches actively utilize compassion, openness, and an awareness of the mental, emotional, spiritual, and physical components of our lives, as well as the healing energy force known as chi, ki, qi, shakti, or kundalini—all names for the feminine aspect of Spirit. I have travelled to India, Japan, Brazil, and Colombia, and have been involved with healing sessions with Ayurvedic doctors, Japanese priests, Native American medicine men, and South American shamans. I've seen firsthand people healed with all of the tools I just mentioned—their physical symptoms released, emotional pain healed, mental confusion clarified, and spiritual disconnection resolved.

The Root of Disease

In modern American culture, we've lost contact with our body's intelligence and given our power away to the authority: the doctor. As a holistic physician, my patients ask me questions they don't ask their conventional doctor. They tell me that they don't speak with their doctors about these issues because the doctors don't have enough time or they think the doctors will think it's not important. My patients also tell me that they feel like a disease and not a whole person when dealing with the traditional Western medical system. Many insurance companies force doctors to spend less and less time with their patients; some contracts allow only ten minutes per patient! No wonder we feel that we can't share important information with the doctor.

Despite these discouraging facts, it is important not to put all the blame on the medical system or even insurance companies, for they are just a small part of the problem. We have disempowered ourselves in a larger way in our day-to-day lives—ceding all our power to the government, the scientific community, religion, and medicine. We have given up the deep feeling of connection, power, and joy related to experiencing God within ourselves and in nature for the promise of finding God somewhere *outside* ourselves. We have ceded control over our own well-being to elected officials, priests, and physicians. We have also lost the connection to—and thus the power of—our intuition, which gives us much better advice about our life than any outside person ever could. This overall disempowered state can lead to conditions such as:

- Physical tension and disease—high blood pressure, back pain, headache, arthritis, irritable bowel, indigestion, etc.

- Emotional imbalances—feelings of loss of control, fear, depression, panic, anger, resentment, and grief at all we have lost by not taking charge.

- Mental disharmony—poor memory, fuzzy thinking, inability to learn from mistakes, and neurotic, obsessive, anxious thinking.

- Spiritual disconnection—loss of connection to Spirit, intuition, and insight.

Thus we end up with more disease and less effective ways to deal with our conditions. When I was in medical school in 1976, when the United States was supposedly on top of the world in terms of power and affluence, our infant mortality rate was twenty-first in the world and we had a higher percentage of chronic disease than most countries. This trend continues. For many diseases, we see that Americans are near the bottom of the list of the afflicted. The more we treat one body while ignoring the others, however, the worse our health becomes as a culture. Even our modern definition of our ills—"disease" rather than "disharmony"—implies we can't get better, that our body has betrayed us and we need outside intervention. On the other hand, *disharmony* implies there is the possibility for our system to heal itself if harmony is regained.

It is time to regain responsibility for our lives by finding and using the best tools to regain the connection to our innate wisdom, courage, and heart. When we start using the tools of proper nutrition, fitness, yoga, breathing, stress reduction, meditation, song, prayer, spiritual connection, and insight, we support all levels of our being. And that's when we find true power and health.

A Different Approach

One warm spring night in 1997, Sierra Bender and I were having dinner in New York City. She had assisted me in my prana yoga teacher training course and shared with me an idea she had for a program for women to help them become more empowered and free in their lives. She was thinking of calling it Boot Camp for Goddesses and was wondering how I felt about the title. She also had a vision of eventually writing an accompanying book containing stories, inspiration, and tools for women to become more empowered in their day-to-day life. With my perspective as a holistic MD, Sierra asked me to be part of the project.

Since then, my good friend and spiritual sister Sierra Bender has taken this vision leaps and bounds beyond what we initially discussed that night. She has dedicated herself to the creation of workshops, programs, and resources to help women find themselves—their power, their beauty, and their creative self—in this ever-constricting world. From her inspiring mission, successful Boot Camp for Goddesses, yoga teacher training, workshops for women and teens, adventures and tours around the world, and her beautiful website, she has touched the lives of thousands of women in a positive way, and in doing so has also affected the lives of many men. I have taken a few of her workshops and have seen the transformation take place firsthand. I feel honored to be a part of this project, one that will bring Sierra's transformational tools from her retreats to women worldwide.

I first met Sierra at Kripalu Center for Yoga & Health in 1996 during a yoga teacher training course. I was leading the anatomy and physiology part of the training program, something I'd done since 1980. I had also directed Kripalu yoga teacher training for eight years and lived at a Kripalu ashram for fifteen years, practicing yoga and meditation daily and working as the resident holistic physician. After that, Sierra took my prana yoga teacher training course in New York City, which I still direct through the Open Center. Sierra was certified as a prana yoga teacher while at the same time traveling to India and becoming immersed in the culture there.

By the time we had that meeting in 1997, we had become good friends. Sierra immersed herself in Native American ways by spending ten years out West and traveling the world, learning healing and ceremonial ways in many indigenous cultures. Her relationship with these tribes and cultures helped her not only heal but also share her teachings and knowledge. Throughout the years, we have spent many hours sharing new tools we were learning for ourselves or teaching others not just yogic but also native and indigenous tools that we have learned from other cultures. We both feel that one of the fundamental problems in our culture is the fact that people, both internally and in terms of relationship, are too tied to a masculine, rational mindset and way of living, which constricts our hearts, wisdom, and creativity. We believe that if people would learn tools to empower themselves to take charge of their lives and connect deeply with Mother Earth, they would then find their inner wisdom, creativity, and love.

From these talks and meditations, Sierra's remarkable 4 Body Fit program evolved, which is the foundation for all her retreats and the core message of this book. Take good care of your spiritual, mental, emotional, and physical bodies, as Sierra calls them, and you will achieve great things—excelling in your quest for inner growth, physical fitness, and personal freedom.

An important factor in any of our healing processes is to put our energy and focus where the true "disease," or imbalance, exists. Often with the importance our culture and medical paradigm places on *physical* medicine, we miss the primary area where the illness or imbalance originated. When we look at all four bodies to find where the primary imbalance occurs and treat this first, we support and rebalance the other bodies, which become better able to heal themselves. Only after we have tried addressing all four bodies should we intervene with the least harmful and most natural treatments first—nutrition, movement, prayer, ritual, and honest expression; then herbal medicine, needles, and therapeutic movement, such as yoga therapy; then, as last resort, stronger herbs, drugs, or surgery.

In our modern culture, though, instead of trying natural cures and rituals *before* moving on to more dangerous interventions as needed, we start with medicines that introduce side effects right away, and if we use natural treatments at all, we only use them as support. By reconnecting to all four bodies and experiencing body intelligence, pure emotional feeling, mental clarity, and spiritual intuition, we regain our faith in nature's healing powers and become empowered through utilizing our own natural healing powers. Sierra's 4 Body Fit approach gives you tools not only to help heal and balance each body but also to regain your connection to the wisdom of each body, so that you find the strength, faith, and patience to allow your being to heal itself first, with outside support secondarily if needed.

As a physician, yoga teacher, father, and male, it has been an amazing journey for me to learn about the feminine experience and psyche from Sierra and her programs. This book not only is an important resource for any woman, but it is just as important for men to become more in touch with the women in their lives and the strength of the feminine within them. As we move deeply into our human evolution during the upcoming years, it feels essential that we all understand the inner and outer feminine more fully to come together in a more real and loving way.

—JEFF MIGDOW, M.D.

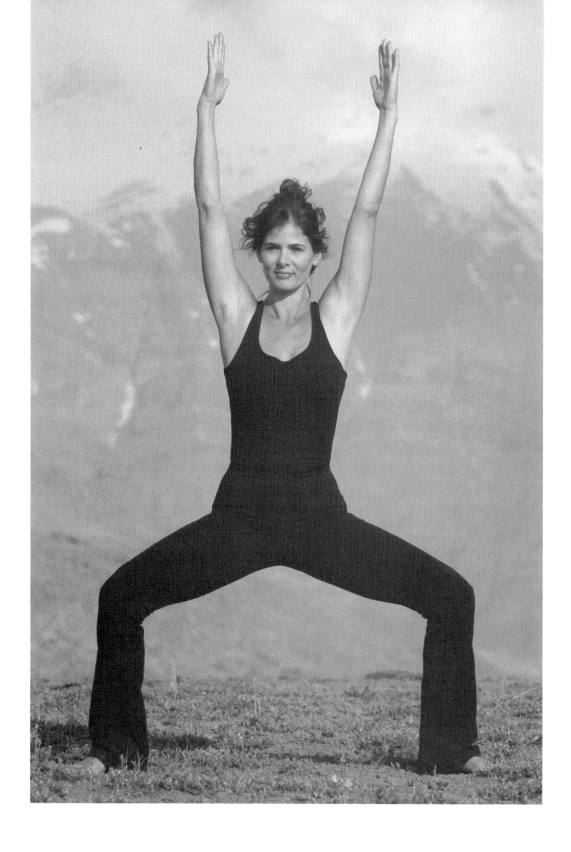

THE AWAKENING

I am in a dark, warm, mysterious place. I feel the coolness of the earth underneath me, and I see hot rocks glistening like stars in the sky as herbs are placed upon them. I can smell the herbs when I inhale and sense their healing power from the inside out. My heart is pounding to the beat of the drum and the sound of magnificent female voices singing their prayers to Mother Earth and Father Sky, asking for forgiveness, praying for those who are sick, and rejoicing and celebrating in their divinity.

As I am engulfed in this beautiful moment, I hear faint crying in the background. I sense a woman behind me, scared and trying not to be heard. I cannot see her, nor can she see me. It is pitch-black in the sweat lodge. I offer my hand to give her comfort and whisper in her ear to lie on Mother Earth. Her face is wet from her tears, and her body shakes from releasing her deepest, darkest fears. I hold her in my arms to ease her pain, rocking her like a baby to help her feel safe. I ask Father Sky and Mother Earth for our prayers to be heard—that this woman, one of their children, is given the strength and perseverance to surrender and let go of what no longer serves her. I whisper my prayers in her ear while she rests her head on my lap. I continue to hold her, to ease her suffering.

She lets out a sigh, followed by a wail from the depths of her soul. Amidst the singing, no one notices her cries, and she becomes overwhelmed by the noise as well as the fear that she is not in control. I ask her to take in deep breaths and to follow my breath. I tell her she needs to focus her mind on her breath alone—nothing else. As she starts to sink into a more meditative and peaceful place, I can feel her muscles starting to surrender.

"Breathe and receive," I tell her. "Your time has come. It's time to let go of unhealthy thoughts, pent-up emotions, and all the toxins that have been taking up space inside you."

I sense that she is drawn by the power of these words and can feel our hearts and souls resonating together. We hear the voices of the other women in the sweat lodge call out from the dark: "One Nation! One God! One Spirit! *Aho*[1]!" Then the door swings open, and light from the fire shines on the faces belonging to those angelic female voices. The brisk night air soothes our skin like a mother's touch. All of my senses are heightened; I've never felt so alive, so clean.

In a sacred ceremony like the one we are in the midst of, we create the space for God to awaken within us—to fill our hearts, bodies, and souls. This is the place of magic, of mystery, and of the unknown. Like the pause between our heartbeats, true healing exists in a place without a sense of time, where everything and anything is possible.

The woman in the sweat lodge was dealing with years of repressed and fractured emotions. She had been going to therapy to deal with a history of sexual abuse as a child. Her therapist had been asking her to recall the incidents, but she couldn't. Her mind couldn't make sense of the horrible events of her past, so I told her to let it all go—to use the sweat lodge as a chance to cleanse herself at the level of her soul. All those suppressed emotions were so embedded in the cellular structure of her body that this sweat lodge experience is a gift, an opportunity to finally rid herself of toxins.

I guided her in this way because I knew her pain. You see, my past is no longer a part of my present. My journey to the present began over a decade ago, when I was thirty years old. Before then, I also suffered through many experiences of abuse. As

---

1   *Aho*, a Native American term used much like the term *namaste*, means to honor Spirit and the light within.

a young woman, I struggled with what this meant and was never able to process it completely. I struggled intensely with my identity, my weight, and my self-esteem. As a result, I ended up with a life that seemed outwardly successful, but really I was traveling on a road to failure. I married too early and found myself in a career as a personal trainer that appeared successful. At the top of my career, I was working with celebrities, professional athletes, CEOs on Wall Street, and the leaders of Fortune 500 companies. Four months into my marriage, I became pregnant. When I discovered my pregnancy, my first reaction was utter happiness—but then reality snuck in. I had a hard time coming to terms with the fact that I was pregnant and that my body was changing. I would talk to the baby and convince myself I was happy, even as my insecurities about being imperfect barreled on full force. The truth was, at times I hated being pregnant. To make matters worse, I was ashamed of feeling that way and had no idea how to handle these confusing emotions.

Unfortunately, I didn't have time to figure it out. On December 23, 1995, I awoke in the middle of the night feeling ill. I felt a growing pressure and a pulling sensation on the inner left side of my pelvis. I ran to the bathroom and threw up. I figured I had morning sickness, but that sensation of pressure wouldn't go away. Eventually, I felt faint and had no idea where I was and no concept of time. My husband called an ambulance on Christmas Eve, and after a long, harrowing experience in the hospital, convulsing, struggling for oxygen, and torn with debilitating pain, my doctor told me I'd suffered a rare ectopic pregnancy that was misdiagnosed in an earlier sonogram. Because of the tubular location of the fetus, it had room to grow up to four months but then ran out of space. The growing pressure ruptured my fallopian tube and uterus completely, pouring eighty percent of my blood into my stomach and requiring four emergency blood transfusions. The doctors did not expect me to survive.

Little did we know, I was a survivor in more ways than one. Technically, I died on the operating table. Although modern medicine saved my life, my near-death experience changed me forever.

Though I may not have realized it at the time, what happened to me in the hospital was a continuation of the issues I had been dealing with all along—and a far cry from the end of my journey. For thirty years, I lived a life that took me further away from my true self, and it took a rare tubular pregnancy and dance with death to bring me back to what I already knew when I was seven years old—that I could hear and heed my intuition, knowing that feelings are real and some things do not need explanation. That I knew how to talk to God, nature, and spirits without any help, and I was not crazy for doing so. That I do not have to tell all my secrets, for I do not have to explain myself to others or defend what I believe. That silence is strength, and listening to my intuition is a way of communicating with the divine.

During my recovery process, my senses and intuition became especially sharp and precise. I could see people's energy. I knew what people were thinking before they spoke. I had a heightened awareness of everything around me and within me. And remarkably, the stiller I became, the more I sensed. It was as if I were constantly watching myself and taking in information about my environment, like a child observing the world for the first time. The most challenging experience of my life blessed me with the gift of seeing and knowing my true purpose. This energy is known in the yoga world as shakti. My kundalini energy had been awakened, and life force emanated from my being. Although I didn't know where I was headed, I knew it was time to leave. I trusted from the depths of my soul that the serenity and wisdom I had experienced on the other side was real, and I was willing to go anywhere on the planet to find it again.

I knew I had to make new choices that supported my new path. Despite the outward success of my job as a personal trainer, internally, I began to understand that my work was perpetuating women's attempts to make themselves conform. I was part of the problem, not part of the solution. It was this realization that laid the foundation for my awakening. I could no longer remain in my marriage; I knew it was soon to be a part of my past. It was time to start searching for my own answers.

My journey led me to the doors of a therapist, an Indian ashram, the Dalai Lama's home, a jail, a sweat lodge, a tipi, and a hut in the Amazon. I rediscovered spirituality, communed the rhythm of the earth, lived with indigenous cultures, found remarkably useful new tools—and in every way created a brand-new worldview, one that is the very foundation of *Goddess to the Core*.

Not everyone has a near-death experience to remind them of their true nature, but many women do get in touch with their power after menopause, when they are done with the hard work of tending to their children. Why does it take us fifty or sixty years to figure out what we knew when we were girls, or when we gave birth and saw the sparkle of God in our baby's eyes, or when we made love and felt close to the god and goddess within?

All of us have unique stories. We have experienced moments of beauty and transcendence and periods of frustration and pain. There are many teachers and healers who are available to give us the information that can help us on our journeys. They are here to offer pieces to the puzzle of our lives, but each one of us has to do our own work. You have to take the first step; you have to take action. Taking action is your responsibility. Taking control of your own destiny is the most powerful form of healing and empowerment. This is self-love, the most powerful energy in the universe. Love is not just an emotion. Love also needs action. *Goddess to the Core* is your resource for turning your love into action.

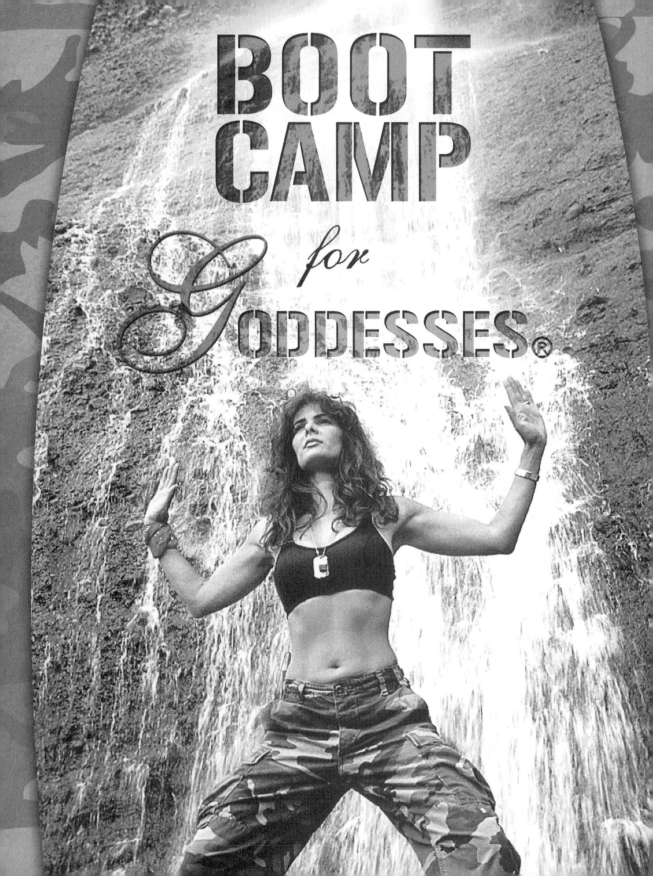

WHAT IS
BOOT CAMP FOR GODDESSES®?

I am the founder of the retreat Boot Camp for Goddesses, an experience that gives you a workout for your body *and* your soul.

Each year, I work with women from all walks of life: CEOs, celebrities, and professional athletes; busy, career-minded women and their daughters; victims of abuse, addicts, and women with eating disorders. No matter what their background is, the majority of women who come to my retreats are feeling disempowered and depleted. The sad part is that they don't even fully realize it—they just know that they have been feeling this way for a long time.

At every Boot Camp for Goddesses, I ask the women, "What do you desire—what are your goals, dreams, and visions? And how do you plan on making them happen?" And every time I do, I see women get frustrated or break into tears because they realize they have lost their way. They have invested all their energy in their kids, their relationships, and their jobs. They have been keeping themselves so busy building other people's kingdoms that they have forgotten their own desires and dreams. And it is a painful realization to see that instead of the fire of action—a healthy and vibrant life force—they quickly see that the only fire they are carrying around is their own anger and rage. Many of the women I meet aren't able to commit to their goals, have problems focusing, and many are even on antidepressants. Although they may have achieved an external level of success, their insides are a mess, because they have been holding themselves back to fit into a prescribed role of what women "should" be instead of blossoming into the women they have the potential to become.

Although we say that women have come a long way, baby, the road we've traveled has led us to become more like men. We have gone so far outside of our true nature that we have become imitation men—masters at swallowing our emotions, fine-tuning our appearance to look younger, and running ourselves ragged keeping work, family, and home running smoothly, all to prove we are reliable, independent, and can do it all. Of course we can do it all—*I am woman: hear me roar, bring home the bacon, and fry it up in the pan*—the question is, do you really *want* to? Our health, children, and relationships are suffering; how can we, as the wealthiest country in the world, have such a high percentage of sexual abuse and addiction issues? And another study shows that the number of Americans using antidepressants doubled in only a decade, while the number seeing psychiatrists continued to fall.[2]

According to the same *USA Today* article, about 10 percent of Americans—or 27 million people—took antidepressants in 2005, the last year for which data was available at the time the study was written. That's about twice the number in 1996, according to a study of nearly 50,000 children and adults in today's *Archives of General Psychiatry*. Yet the majority weren't being treated for depression. Half of those taking antidepressants used them for back pain, nerve pain, fatigue, sleep difficulties, or other problems, the study says.[3]

"Doctors are now medicating unhappiness," said Dr. Ronald Dworkin, a Maryland anesthesiologist and senior fellow at the Hudson Institute. "Too many people take drugs when they really need to be making changes in their lives."[4] According to this government study, antidepressants have become the most commonly prescribed drugs in the United States.[5] In its study, the U.S. Centers for Disease Control and Prevention looked

2   See http://www.usatoday.com/news/health/2009-08-03-antidepressants_N.htm.

3   Ibid.

4   See http://www.bio-medicine.org/medicine%2Dnews/Americans%2DBloated%2DOn%2D%2D Happy%2DPills%2D23608%2D1.

5   Ibid.

at 2.4 billion drugs prescribed in visits to doctors and hospitals in 2005. Of those, 118 million were for antidepressants.[6] Adult use of antidepressants almost tripled between the periods 1988–1994 and 1999–2000.[7]

Consider these sobering statistics:

- Between 1995 and 2002, the most recent year for which statistics are available, the use of antidepressants rose 48 percent.[8]

- The Department of Health and Human Services released a survey estimating that child abuse and neglect in the United States nearly doubled during the years between 1986 and 1993.[9]

- Between 100 and 140 million girls and women in the world have undergone some form of female genital mutilation. In sub-Saharan Africa, Egypt, and the Sudan, 3 million girls and women are subjected to genital mutilation every year.[10]

- One in four girls is sexually assaulted before the age of eighteen.[11]

- One out of every six American women has been the victim of an attempted or completed rape in their lifetime.[12]

- Most perpetrators of sexual violence are men. Among acts of sexual violence committed against women eighteen and older, 100 percent of rapes, 92 percent of physical assaults, and 97 percent of stalking acts were perpetrated by men.[13]

---

6   Ibid.

7   Ibid.

8   Ibid.

9   See http://www.prevent-abuse-now.com/stats.htm.

10   See http://www.un.org/apps/news/story.asp?NewsID=20225&Cr=child&Cr1.

11   See http://www.darkness2light.org/KnowAbout/statistics_2.asp.

12   See http://www.fhsu.edu/kellycenter/counseling/statistics.shtml.

13   See http://www.ruralwomyn.net/domvio_cultural.html.

Despite all the progress we've made since the days when women couldn't vote or own property, women still earn less than men and are still taught to look pretty, be nice, and not take up too much space. If you don't believe that women have learned to diminish themselves, look around the next time you are in a group of women—how many of them have their arms folded over their stomachs, their legs crossed, and their chests shrunken, as if they were trying to squeeze themselves into an invisible box? Either that or you see women who are overly aggressive or manipulative with their sexuality.

If you look at the messages we receive from the world around us, you can see how women have learned to minimize their presence. The word *feminine* has come to mean soft, loving, warm, and docile—all adjectives with no action behind them. Fitness in our society isn't about developing a better relationship with your body; it's a means of coaxing your body to look more like some unattainable ideal or to punish yourself if you don't live up to that ideal. Even yoga, with its ultimate goal of joining mind and body, has been forced into service as a means of selling cute yoga pants and designer mats. Our society prizes beauty but defines it as looking appealing by any means necessary—whether it be surgery, starvation, prescription medication, or slathering our bodies in chemicals. And the only kind of power we recognize is the power *over* others—a typically patriarchal definition of power. Power from *within* is either overlooked completely or not valued.

Yet as tempting as it may be to blame society, the media, religion, or even our parents, the fact is that we women are accomplices in our own disempowerment. We distract ourselves with drama, addiction, and bad habits to keep our mind and feelings numb to our pain. In the long run, these distractions waste our precious energy and time, take us further away from our spiritual selves, and create stress, which in turn kicks off a downward spiral—we blame others for whatever is triggering our stress and thereby assume the role of victim. *Victim* comes from the Latin *victima,* which means "sacrifice." Are you sacrificing yourself?

Approaching life as a victim hinders us from taking action. It makes us willing participants in our own *dis*-ease. Stress takes up so much of our attention that we are losing all self-awareness and therefore the ability to heal ourselves. We do have a choice. We don't have to accept these cultural mandates as our destiny. In fact, we have an imperative to reclaim beauty, fitness, power, and femininity for ourselves.

Bringing Boot Camp Home to You

Fortunately, there are tools from cultures all over the world that we can use to break the cycle of stress, upset, and disconnect from our core selves, bringing us greater well-being. My mission is to share these tools with you and to teach you how to create what you desire, require, and deserve.

Goddess to the Core brings the boot camp experience home so you can live it on a regular basis. The experience, as outlined in this book, starts on the inside and works its way out, redefining power, beauty, and fitness as we go. By starting the journey, you will reclaim the power of your feminine essence. You will learn how to face your fears head-on; find answers to why you are not getting what you desire, require, and deserve; and discover tools to put yourself first, without forgetting others, to truly rejoice in your own skin. You will claim your place as a strong, knowing, intuitive, and powerful goddess.

Empowerment is derived from a Greek word that means pulling forth what is already within you. *Goddess to the Core* will pull the power, beauty, mystery, and magic out of you. Don't get me wrong: I will make you sweat, but it's just as important to the process that you also laugh and shed some tears. In the process, you will move from fear and discomfort to an open, intuitive space where you can ask questions and find answers. You will learn what I call the other side of power—surrendering, the power to let go of what doesn't serve you, so that your true self has room and space to grow. You will be able to relinquish old habits, patterns, beliefs, resentments, and worries once and for all, making room for creativity, change, and abundance. This action could affect all aspects of your life and help you find a new job, strengthen your loving relationships, discover your purpose, know your self-worth, heal old habits, and even find peace.

I cannot promise this process will be easy. In fact, it can be downright painful to give up the beliefs, habits, and attitudes that no longer serve you. After all, you have likely been carrying these thoughts around for as long as you can remember. You have become comfortable with them. Letting them go can be incredibly scary. But in order to cross over to the other side of power, you have to take a leap. Fear and faith are both invisible and intangible, yet it takes more guts to choose faith over fear.

Goddess to the Core will help you give birth to your goddess self. Part physical workout, part yoga practice, part spiritual reflection, *Goddess to the Core* will help you achieve ultimate well-being. I am the midwife in the process, ushering you between the world of your past and your new reality. It's a journey that will challenge and heal all aspects of your being.

Discovering the goddess in your core (and yes, you are a goddess) is about treating yourself as a vibrant, healthy, multidimensional being. Today, living as we do in developed areas, often disconnected from spirituality and nature, caring for our families and running here and there, from errand to appointment and home again to cook, clean, and pay the bills, it's all too easy to forget that there is so much more to life than what we see on the physical plane.

I teach women to discover all four planes of existence—spiritual, mental, emotional, and physical—a process that leads to enlightenment, integration, and wholeness. When we learn how to keep all four planes of our existence fit, we become healthier, happier, and better able to lead our families, friends, and communities to do the same for themselves.

I call this process 4 Body Fit as a constant reminder to you that you are a multidimensional, vibrant being. 4 Body Fit is the foundation of my work—it is the basis for Boot Camp for Goddesses and the foundation of this book.

The first step in our journey is to understand that just because we don't comprehend or can't see something doesn't mean it doesn't exist. We all know we have a physical body. It is the structure that contains our organs and keeps us alive and functioning. The nervous, circulatory, respiratory, endocrine, and other systems work as a team to coordinate balance and harmony in the physical body and keep us healthy. But even though we were all taught in basic science that without the heart pumping blood and the lungs taking in oxygen we could not exist, how do we really know this information to be true? We trust that scientists and the medical field know more than we do—and in most cases they do if we are dealing with only one dimension: the physical body. But ask a spiritual leader the same question, and you might discover a very different answer; who is to say who is right?

How many times have you thought, sensed, or felt something was physically wrong with you, only to go through a series of tests at the doctor's office and be told that your problem is stress related or possibly just in your mind. Then the manifestation comes weeks or months later, perhaps as a cyst, a lump, a kidney infection, maybe a heart murmur—whatever it is, hopefully it appears before it is life threatening. It's no coincidence that you knew something was wrong with your body before anyone else was able to see it. I call this underrated phenomenon *body intelligence.*

Each body has its own intelligence. Intuition, pain, hunger, feelings, instincts, needs, wants, joy, desires, love—all these things are your spiritual, mental, emotional, and physical wisdom. So, while the physical body literally holds us together, the demise of the spiritual, mental, or emotional body is no less debilitating or painful, even though it is sometimes harder to see.

As a culture, we are taught to take care of our physical body, often to the detriment of the other three bodies. Taking care of the emotional, spiritual, and mental bodies is no less important than taking care of the physical body. And there are many different sources out there to help you do so: psychologists, psychiatrists, preachers, doctors, personal trainers, priests, artists, musicians, and writers—all of these people are healers in their chosen field. You need to rely on their resources, create your own, and learn how to nurture, feed, and "treat" your emotional, spiritual, and mental body as much as your physical body.

When women come to boot camp, I help them realize the health benefits of awakening and maintaining all four of their bodies. One woman will come looking for spiritual reconnection and cannot understand why she feels so lost spiritually. Another woman will come because of a high-end job in the corporate world, hoping to find ways of relieving mental stress. Another woman will come because she is looking to rebuild her confidence emotionally after a bad relationship. And another woman will come to rebuild herself physically because she has kids and many demands at home and is not feeling comfortable in her body. Remarkably, it doesn't matter which angle you come at it. To get into "shape," you must exercise all four bodies to be truly fit. This is a workout plan that exercises all four aspects of being, that gets to the main point, working to your goal: a balanced being who is fit inside and out.

How Four-Body Fitness Helps You Grow

SPIRITUALLY: Integrates the flow of physical, emotional, and mental energies. Four-body fitness is the path to inner knowing and the way to understanding. Through this practice, you will come to realize the true essence of your divine nature.

MENTALLY: Teaches the discipline of silence and stillness, allowing the mind and heart to evaluate and reflect instead of merely reacting.

EMOTIONALLY: Creates a union between the body, breath, and emotions. The breath is the catalyst that deepens emotional intelligence and permits the body's stored cellular memory to physically release, thus creating a stronger sense of self and of inner peace.

PHYSICALLY: Builds the foundation of the physical body by placing equal emphasis on strength and suppleness. It gives stability to the skeletal system and creates a more flexible muscular system.

The following chapters teach you everything you need to know about balancing your four bodies:

- What are the four bodies?
- How do I connect to them?
- How do I cleanse them?
- How do I build the muscles of each body?
- How do I get energy from them?
- How do I heal them?
- How do they connect to nature?

Although the four bodies are separate and distinct planes of existence, they are also all interconnected. Imagine four different masses of energy, each one progressively denser. They are laid on top of each other, and they are all flowing and pulsating through, in, and throughout each other. It is best described in yogic philosophy: the spiritual body is the subtlest, with the quickest vibration that emerged from the source of all life. Then, as the vibration slowed, the energy became more solid and formed the mental body. The next body to form was the emotional body, which is denser still than the mental body. And finally, the energy grew more solid and vibrated more slowly to form the physical body.

The bodies range from the tangible to the intangible—from the physical to the auric (emotional), astral (mental), and invisible (spiritual). The spiritual body is a flash of inspiration, the mental body is the understanding of the inspiration, the emotional body is the feelings that the understanding elicits, and the physical is the manifestation of the inspiration.

In yoga, we often hear teachers say how the spirit is higher than our body, mind, or emotions. In education, the mind is supreme. In the arts, emotion rules. And in athletics, the physical body is the star of the show. But when we begin to believe that one aspect of us is more important than another, we create internal tension around those bodies we aren't quite as in tune with, which leads to physical tension, emotional upset, mental agitation, and spiritual disconnection. In time, this can become dis-ease such as high blood pressure, fibromyalgia, anxiety, depression, negativity, anger toward self and others, and becoming out of touch with the deeper parts of yourself.

The Way to Reunification

This book contains tools that are designed to challenge, work, heal, and treat all four bodies. The goal is to create suppleness, flexibility, balance, focus, and full range of motion in all four bodies. And in doing so, we can rehabilitate, recycle, reprogram, and re-energize your entire being. All the answers you need to change your life for the better are within you; you just don't recognize them…*yet*.

No matter what your fitness level or whether or not you consider yourself a spiritual person, my program will take you full circle, helping you experience the full spectrum of human experience and teaching you the importance of being present in your own body. You'll learn to listen to your body's natural wisdom; strengthen its healing capacity; challenge yourself emotionally, physically, spiritually, and mentally; and meet fears head-on. You'll be stronger for it, and you'll be better able to recover and learn from setbacks.

Working with your four bodies requires a commitment to creating harmony and balance within yourself. It takes discipline to stop, look, listen, and feel. And it can feel like a sacrifice to make time to retreat, meditate, and pray, to move your attention inward so you can gain insight and find the strength to go forward on your path. But as a result of this process, you will move from a scared, uncomfortable place to an open, intuitive space where you can ask questions and find answers.

The Four-Body Approach Throughout History

The number four has an important place in the history of our cultures and healing systems:

- The four directions most cultures use to describe movement and space—north, south, east, and west.

- The four seasons: spring, summer, fall, and winter.

- The four elements of the Greeks and other cultures, which describe the aspects of nature in all of her forms: fire, air, water, and earth.

- The four horses of the Apocalypse in Revelation, which represent destruction of all darkness and negativity in all four bodies in all four corners of the world.

- The four basic sheaths in yoga philosophy and Ayurvedic medicine, which explain the levels of our true infinite nature: intuitive, rational, energetic, and physical. The fifth and most subtle sheath is the bliss sheath, which is the experience we have when the other four bodies are healthy and in balance.

- The four stages of life: childhood, young adult/parent, middle age/grandparent, and elder/wise person.

- The four colors of race: red (Native), black (African American), white (Caucasian), and yellow (Eastern Asian).

- It is a Native American teaching that we have four generations before us, alive or passed over, that have guided us, healed us, and given us gifts as much as genetic dysfunctions that we shift through each generation by healing and/or teaching others the tribal laws of life as the natives know it.

Imagine, hope, and reach for your full potential. Become who you truly are. Find your true nature. This is the foundation of the self-love, self-respect, self-esteem, courage, worthiness, and natural wisdom that exists within each of us. When we've mastered this natural state of being, we've found our true nature. Remember, each of us is a creation of God, and our lives are evidence of the god within each of us.

Before we go into all the specific tools to awaken each of your bodies, we need to look at how we got into this whole mess in the first place.

ℱour-body case studies

A medical perspective from Jeff Migdow, M.D.

Here are two examples from my practice on how bringing balance to one body brings health and harmony back to all four bodies.

Case Study No. 1:

A man in his forties saw me for high blood pressure. Although he was being treated with medication, his blood pressure wasn't normalizing. When he saw me for holistic treatment, we explored all his bodies and came to see the primary problem was actually in his mind. He was very upset with the state of the world—crime, poverty, wars, and the lack of compassion many governments displayed toward their people. He was obsessed with staying caught up on these issues. He watched the news constantly, increasing his mental tension all day.

We focused on his mental body to help calm his mind through breathing and relaxation techniques, meditation, commitment to watching the news only once a day, and shifting his mental framework to focus on the positives that occurred during the day to create a more balanced mental perspective. After a few months, he had a healthier attitude and felt happier in general. He was able to put more energy into the issues he truly wanted to help transform. And physically, his blood pressure lowered to a normal range.

Because we took the time to explore all four bodies, we were able to pinpoint his primary imbalance. Even though he came to me to treat a physical disease, his treatment was strengthening his mental body in a healthy way. Through this four-body approach, his blood pressure came down to normal range, but more importantly, he became a healthier, happier, calmer person, and he still is today.

When one or more of the bodies are weaker or overworked, this creates a feeling of fragmentation. This fragmentation pulls the other bodies out of alignment with each other, therefore creating an overall imbalance, leading to disease. However, when we bring balance and alignment to all four bodies, we create overall health spiritually, mentally, emotionally, and physically.

Case Study No. 2:

I once saw a woman in her sixties who was suffering from severe arthritis, anxiety, and depression. She had seen a conventional doctor and psychiatrist and had been on painkillers for her arthritis and medicines for her anxiety and depression for decades, yet her symptoms remained.

During her first few sessions with me, we discussed all the aspects of her life, and I discovered that she had been sexually and physically abused as a child. It was clear that these experiences had taken up residence in her spiritual body, manifesting as a lack of trust, a lack of a relationship with any form of God, and an inability to hear her intuition. From these insights, we realized that her lack of faith and trust—a strong weakness in her spiritual body—had led to her anxiety and depression. Any situation where she needed to depend on another human would set off a near-panic response. The depression was a direct outcome of feeling helpless and hopeless for decades. The arthritis was secondary to severe tension in the structure of her body, as it was holding on for dear life against the unknown shifts and changes of life and a lack of stretching and exercise due to the fear that if she used her body too much, she would have a heart attack and die. She was in a chronically constricted state.

Because she could see how her patterns, created over fifty years before, had negatively impacted all four of her bodies, she committed to going through the work of rebuilding her faith and trust in life, her connection to Spirit, and her inner knowing. We did this over the next few months by helping her see all the wonderful events that had occurred in her life since she was in her twenties—that, in fact, life had taken good care of her the past forty years, and there was much to be grateful for and hopeful about. This didn't negate the experience of her abuse. In fact, because she felt more hopeful and open, we explored the childhood abuse more deeply than she had in the past and came to the realization that although she would never forget the deep pain from her childhood, her experience since then had truly balanced things out. She could now experience the old feelings without being a victim to them. She also started a walking and yoga practice. As a result, she was able to focus on the present and enjoy what she had now much more fully.

She went totally off her anti-anxiety medicine, greatly decreased her anti-depressants, and lowered her pain medication. She had much less physical pain and was happier, clearer, and more connected to her inner source than she had been since she was a young child. During our last appointment, she remarked how these changes had only occurred due to our shifting of focus from the physical and emotional bodies to the spiritual, where the main imbalance was occurring.

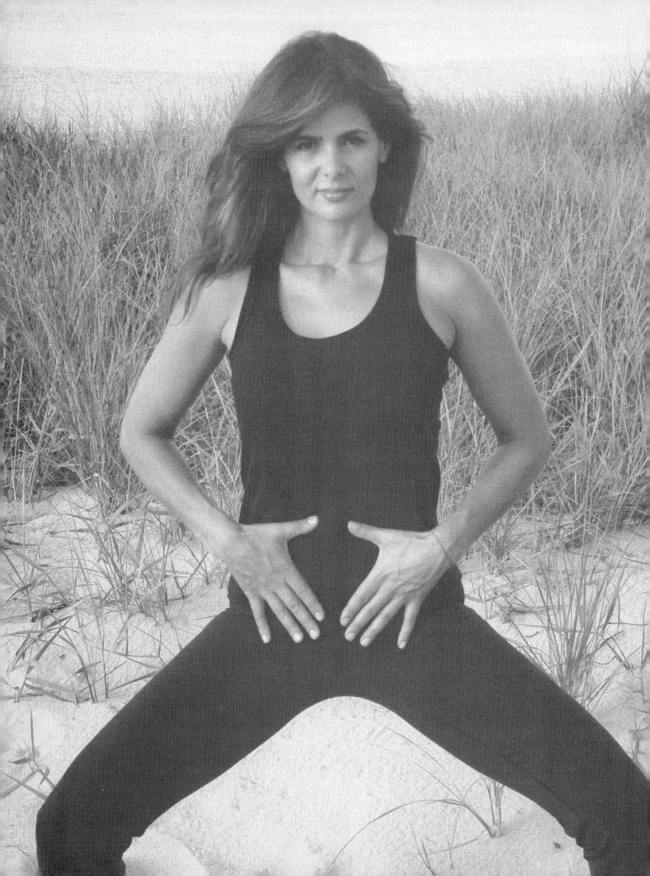

Chapter 1

WHERE WE LOST OUR CORE

The Source of Women's Anger

It didn't take me long to realize girls were treated differently than boys. When I was seven years old, I was subjected to a lot of rules that were different than the rules my brothers and the neighborhood boys had to follow. I was carefully told to be home by dark, to not draw attention to myself or talk to strangers. It felt so unfair. I wanted to act with trust and express myself to my fullest potential, yet these warnings made me afraid that I would get hurt by someone or something if I spent time with boys, walked home alone, or stayed out late at night. I did not know about sex yet, but I had some idea that boys and men could hurt me and that the world was unsafe for a girl. This was when the belief that men had more power than women was first instilled in me, and that the world was not a level playing field. I was sad I could not be as free as the boys, and then, as much as it does now, made me angry.

Based on the thousands of women I have worked with in my retreats, I can attest that I am by no means the only woman who carries around this innate, deep feeling of something akin to anger—something we can't easily pinpoint but that challenges our very lives. In many cases, the women I've worked with have had a history of challenges, struggles, or even abuse that keeps them from digging deep into and realizing their core dreams. It is painful to see that instead of the fire of action—a healthy and vibrant force—the only fire they are carrying around is their own frustration, anger, and rage. Women are still subjected to the shadow of the old forms of oppression. It wasn't that long ago that a woman's place was in the home, cleaning and making dinner. If she worked, it was only in one of a few chosen fields, and marriage and child-rearing were considered the most obvious signs of her success. It's amazing how far we have evolved since then, but we still have a lot more evolving to do.

On a global level, the picture is more grim than it is in the United States. Why is it that men are the ones who create most of the violence in the world, yet women are punished for it by having to stay in at night for fear of being raped, molested, kidnapped, or killed? Rape is considered a weapon of war. To destroy a culture, a common tactic is to rape the women in order to contaminate the lineage and unravel the community. The women who have been raped can no longer go back to their families, because they are considered a disgrace to their families.

In India, if there is not enough money in the home, girls do not go to school. Only boys are educated, while the girls stay at home to work with their mothers or are married at such a young age that they essentially become slaves. Many girls die of starvation or disease, or are killed before they reach their teenage years. When I travelled to India in 1997, I learned that girl fetuses were aborted, because girls, just another mouth to feed, were not seen to be as valuable as boys. The hair on the back of my neck stood up, and I felt a surge of anger climb up my spine. I was empowered to explore what I could do to stop this. I recognized that not only was this a crime against women in India, it was a blow to all women around the world. The anger it unleashed gave me the energy to take action, and although I didn't know it at the time, this anger made me confront my own issues and brought my ideas for Boot Camp for Goddesses to the forefront.

To think that these horrible crimes do not affect women as a whole is irresponsible and offensive. This violence leads to the slow death of a woman's spirit and soul in a global sense. All women are sisters, and all sisters are goddesses, no matter where we live. We have been so conditioned and numb to this violence toward women that we do not realize how it has affected us, our children, our relationships, and the earth. The concept of being feminine has been distorted in the name of diluting our power and essence so that others can benefit from our losses, such as businesses making money selling us a houseful of products that will allegedly make us feel beautiful and worthy again.

Of course we all want to be beautiful, healthy, and vibrant, but at what cost? And who is defining what is fit, healthy, and beautiful? Corporations, medical establishments, and media constantly reinforce the idea that if we are not pretty, we aren't worthy of attention, love, or success. Or if we have children, we have no worth, because motherhood is not valued as a full-time job. Or if we age, our partners will no longer want us and will leave us for a younger woman.

Is it any wonder why eating disorders, drug problems, and depression are so prevalent in women and girls? The needier and less self-contained we are, the more these industries stand to make off of us. We are searching for validation from the outside in because, as a whole, we women have lost touch with our own worth. We have been taught since we were little girls to love others before ourselves. We are conditioned to give our love away selflessly, but we do not recognize that when we do this, we also give up our own desires, dreams, and, most of all, our health. We become last on our own list. We tell ourselves that giving ourselves selflessly to taking care of others is the only way to prove that we love them unconditionally. Ladies, I've got news for you: this is codependence, not love.

If you find yourself inexplicably frustrated or angry on a deep soul level, there is nothing wrong with you. You probably have had many experiences just like mine as a young girl and have never been taught what to do with your feelings. We have kept our rage so suppressed that we are shocked and scared when it shows its ugly head. And when we express this anger to those closest to us—particularly the men we love—it is too ugly or too deep for them to understand. They call us crazy and hysterical, because they forget or cannot fathom that women as a whole have been denied freedoms and treated as second class for thousands of years.

The Story of Lilith

Let me tell you the story of how I finally discovered the words to explain my own anger and made a choice to put it to use instead of being consumed by it.

When I was engaged to a Jewish man, I decided to convert to Judaism because I wanted our children to grow up with one religion. Although I was brought up Catholic, as a child I never liked the idea of fearing God. (It's funny how I knew even as a young girl that God was not something to be feared.) I started attending Hebrew school and fell in love with the Jewish religion and the stories I learned about all the rituals and how the woman had a certain role in each ceremony. As I explored Hebrew studies, it was re-learning the story of Adam and Eve that introduced me to my own inner divinity. As a Catholic, my understanding of the story of Adam and Eve was simple: Eve bit the apple, and all hell broke loose. It was Eve who brought sin to the world and suffering to all humankind. This is pretty heavy stuff for a young girl to be taught as God's honest truth. The Hebrew version of Adam and Eve made more sense to my ears and to my heart, and it gave me a clue about where some of my anger might be coming from. When I tell this story to other women, a light bulb goes off, and it all rings true for them too. Everything starts to shift.

In truth, the Adam and Eve parable we are taught as children is only part two of the story. In part one, there is also a woman named Lilith. Lilith is Adam's first partner. But because she wants to be equal to Adam, Lilith refuses to lie beneath him. She confronts both Adam and God, and in the end she leaves Adam, defying patriarchy, refusing to take a submissive sexual posture, and rejecting marriage altogether because it would require her to live under Adam's authority. Lilith becomes what all tyrants fear: a person who is aware that she is enslaved. She then transforms herself into a snake and hides in a tree in the garden of good and evil.

When Adam asks God for a woman to lie beneath him, he offers his rib to God and is rewarded with Eve, a beautiful young maiden who naturally will agree to lie beneath him, since she is made from his body. Lilith, disguised as a snake, befriends Eve and whispers into her ear about the ways of the universe. Empowered by Lilith's wisdom, Eve eats the apple, which represents sweetness and oneness with God and nature—in other words, enlightenment.

In ancient times, men feared Lilith because she knew the power of her sexuality, and she knew that her sexuality had power over men. Women, who have been molded to follow the example of submissive Eve, also fear Lilith because of the power she holds. But this version of the myth shows that Lilith is not an enemy of humankind. She holds the ancient fruit of knowledge, the secrets of our deepest sexual and spiritual nature, and she is willing to offer this fruit to us, the nectar of this truth.

Lilith means "the night," and she embodies the emotional and spiritual aspects of darkness: terror, sensuality, wisdom, and unbridled freedom. More recently, she has come to represent the freedom of feminist women who no longer want to be "good girls." Not surprisingly, Lilith has become the most notorious demon in Jewish tradition. This persona grew, in part, out of repression: repression of sexuality, repression of the freedom of women, and repression of the following question: *What if I left it all behind?* As women as a whole wake up to their own mistreatment and ask questions about sex, freedom, and choice, Lilith becomes a complex, beautiful representation of our own desires.

Eve is the intuitive, feminine aspect of humanity. Adam is the linear, masculine quality. The apple is the knowledge that we are all divine and connected to each other through our relationship to Mother Earth. The snake is the spiritual energy that yogis call kundalini or shakti. Within this scenario, we can see that our spiritual energy naturally supplies our intuitive side with the knowledge of the true nature of reality. However, when our intuitive side shares this knowledge with our linear, calculating side, shame and fear always result. Rather than accepting that oneness of reality and gratefully merging with it, our masculine self becomes ashamed and afraid of this ultimate gift and separates from the truth by ignoring this energy and forcing the feminine to leave the garden with him. What's worse, he blames the feminine—and woman is forever tainted as the cause of original sin.

When we accepted the shame of Adam and the guilt of Eve, not only did we lose the chance to experience the true reality of total connectedness—otherwise known as paradise—we were also made to feel ashamed for our hunger for knowledge. We need to rewrite the story and allow our male side to embrace the knowledge of feminine intuition. Only then do we learn how to experience our true selves, with no guilt or shame. The power that Eve and Lilith embody is within every woman, waiting to come into fruition as we age.

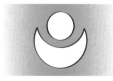

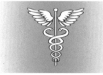

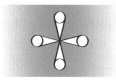

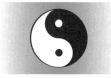

*Symbols from top to bottom: Goddess,
caduceus, yin/yang, ankh, and four elements.*

What Symbols Teach Us

Ancient shamans knew that in order to survive and thrive, they needed to create balance between the masculine and feminine energies. The symbols of the ancient world illustrate this law of energy and life. Stories, myths, and fables from thousands of years ago have instilled long-lasting meaning in our cultures.

On page 6 of this book, I am pictured in front of a waterfall in a posture that represents the universal symbol for Goddess, one of the oldest symbols of humankind. The Goddess's arms raise up toward the sky; her breasts are full and her body is bountiful, reflecting the fertility and strength of Mother Earth. She is round yet firm in her being, giving as well as receptive to the universe's abundance and power.

In the picture by the waterfall, my heart is open to the universe, my arms are pointing up to Father Sky for strength and growth, and my feet are firmly planted on the earth. I claim my space, my birthright on this planet, and know that earth sustains me and holds me, while sky provides me the sunlight and the life force to exist and thrive. This photo was taken near a 300-foot waterfall nestled deep in the wilderness of the Colorado Mountains on the Continental Divide at 12,000 feet above sea level. It was a beautiful summer day, the view was amazing, and suddenly it started to hail. I felt connected to the entire universe at that moment and felt energy move through me like a bolt of lightning.

Unfortunately, most of us are disconnected from the transformative power of these ancient symbols. Going back to the story of Adam, Lilith, and Eve, most of us are taught that the snake is a symbol to fear—it is seen as scary, mischievous, and poisonous. But in Eastern philosophy, the snake is a representation of kundalini, the ball of vital energy that sits in the root chakra, awaiting a trigger to rise and bring enlightenment. Native Americans look at the snake as the closest being to Mother Earth and a metaphor for transmutation, transformation, shedding your skin, and getting rid of your weaknesses and turning them into strengths. The South American natives believe the snake is the symbol of healing. There are clues in our own society that point to these older, deeper views of snake symbolism, particularly the medical symbol known as the caduceus.

The caduceus is based on an Egyptian symbol representing the balance of the male and female and reaching toward God and enlightenment. The two snakes represent the male and female energies, and the sword represents the spinal cord. It's just another example of how the deeper truth exists if you know where and how to look for it.

Circles and crosses are some of the first symbols drawn by children of all cultures. A cross inside a circle is one of the oldest and most widespread of symbols in the Western world. It often stood for the sun and the tree of life. It is comparable to the yin/yang symbol of the Eastern world.

The original cross was the Egyptian ankh—a cross with a circle on the top. The circle represented the female, and the stem represented the male. The horizontal line in the cross represents both male and female forces uniting. The ankh as a whole is a hieroglyph that was used to represent life and death, male and female, and sexual union.

Another widespread symbol that combined the cross and the circle was the four-element symbol. The vertical and horizontal lines represent the male energy; the circles, the female. The funnel mimics a chakra and the spiral of DNA.

Over the years, we have been all but cut off from the immense power that these ancient symbols convey. What's worse, when the patriarchal Christian systems took over, they changed all the symbols in order to squelch the feminine aspect of God. They changed the ancient name for Mother Earth in the Gaelic, Druid, and Celtic traditions from Gaea to Gaia. *E* is a female vowel, a neverending circle, while the linear *I* represents the male. When Christians took over, everything that represented the feminine essence of spirit was taken out of plain view. In doing so, they changed words, symbols, and meanings to best suit the patriarchal system they believed in. The circle was no longer a part of the cross. The Roman emperor Constantine even made the cross a symbol of punishment and death, forming it out of a sword and a spear. For example, the Mexicans called Mother Earth *Tonantzin Tlalli*, meaning "Revered Mother Earth." The natives of the Andes called Mother Earth *Pachamama*—*mama* meaning "mother" and *pacha* meaning "world, space-time, and the universe." After the Spanish Christian conquest of South America, however, many of these Mother Earth symbols were replaced by Christianity's Virgin Mary.

Of all the knowledge we have—religious, historical, political, moral—do you ever wonder where it came from? Or do you follow it because you are told to? We are so trained to trust the media, historians, teachers, and even our parents, because we believe they are more knowledgeable than we are. In some cases they may be, but as we evolve as a race, our truth has to evolve as well. History—"his story"—has given us a one-sided perspective. If you look more closely, you can see an alternative version of history and reality. You simply have to choose to look.

The Influence of Religion

Most of us were taught the myth that God is a man. This is where religion has fundamentally failed and damaged us. It is one of the world's greatest shames that we have only half the equation of God. We need the other half—the Goddess, or the feminine aspect of God—in order to be whole, in order to achieve our fullest expression and balance of life. The word *goddess* is derived from the word *god*; goddess is the feminine essence of god. The goddess Durga is also known as Devi to the Indians and Diva to the Italians, from the Latin word *diva*, meaning "goddess," the feminine version of *divus*, meaning "god."

Here is evidence of how organized religion has stifled women throughout history. Consider these quotes from the Bible:

- "For the man is not of the woman, but the woman of man. Neither was the man created for the woman but the woman for man." (1 Cor. 11:8–9)

- "I permit no woman to have authority over men. She is to be silent." (1 Timothy 2:12)

- "Wives, be subject to your husbands, as to the Lord." (Ephesians 5:22)

These are just a few of the many texts present in the sacred scriptures of the Judeo-Christian tradition that have been used over the centuries to denigrate women, assign them second-class positions, and prevent them from exercising such natural rights of citizenship as voting, becoming educated, and assuming roles of religious leadership. Every advance that women have made has had to fight against these biblical definitions and deformations. The fact that God has been envisioned in the Judeo-Christian tradition almost exclusively as a male has only added fuel to the fires of oppression, and today the Christian church remains the major bulwark of patriarchy.

Religious negativity toward women, however, is not limited to the Judeo-Christian tradition: it appears in other non-Western cultures and most of the great religions of the world. In a sacred text of the Hindus, we are told: "It is the highest duty of woman to immolate herself after her husband's death." In another Hindu text, we read: "Women are to be debarred from being competent students of the Vedas [sacred Hindu scripture]." In the laws of Manu, the Hindu creator of humankind, we read: "In childhood, a female is subject to her father. In youth, a female is subject to her husband. When her Lord is dead, she shall be subject to her sons. A women must never be independent."

In Buddhism, one is reborn a woman because of one's bad karma. Buddhist prayers include: "I pray that I may be reborn a male in a future existence."

From a book of Jewish prayers, Jewish men are taught to say: "Blessed be the god who has not created me a heathen, a slave, or a woman." Talmudic writers added: "It would be better to burn the words of Torah than to entrust them to a woman."

In the Muslim Qu'ran (Koran), we learn that the woman is regarded as "half a man" and that forgetfulness overcomes the woman, who is inherently weaker in "rational judgment."

Plato, in the *Republic*, records Socrates as saying: "Do you know anything at all practiced among mankind in which the male sex is not far better than the female?" Xenophon stated that "the ideal woman should see as little as possible, hear as little as possible, and ask as little as possible."

Even in magazines such as *Housekeeping Monthly* there was the "Good Wife's Guide," from May 13, 1955. Let me share some guidelines that our ancestors not so long ago had to follow. These will help you tap into the innate anger over what our mothers and grandmothers had to endure:

> "A good wife always knows her place. Don't complain if he's late for dinner or even if he stays out all night. Count this as minor compared to what he might have gone through that day.
>
> Arrange his pillow and offer to take off his shoes. Speak in a low, soothing, and pleasant voice.
>
> Don't ever ask him questions about his actions or question his judgment or integrity. Remember: he is the master of the house, and as such will always exercise his will with fairness and truthfulness. You have no right to question him.
>
> Listen to him. You may have a dozen important things to tell him, but the moment of his arrival is not the time. Let him talk first—remember, his topics of conversation are more important than yours."

These are only some of the guidelines; there are many more. When I read this to a group, the oldest goddess, the wisewoman of the group, who was eighty-seven years old, laughed and said to the group, "I do not have to read this; I lived it, honey." So you can have compassion for the women who were handcuffed by the injustice of these beliefs.

And we wonder where our innate anger comes from! Do not think some of these beliefs were not handed down to you. It is the very reason why most mothers and daughters have problems in their relationships.

The beliefs may have changed as we evolved as women, but the core of the beliefs is still in our lineage. We have become smarter, more independent, and better able to fight the injustice, yet deep inside our core, these original seeds lie dormant. They are embedded deep in our souls and have deadened the feminine essence of Spirit and ourselves.

As much as we have seemingly overcome so many of these negative influences, the denigration of women is deeply wrapped up in our history. It's been with us so long that many of us don't even see it anymore. Not only are women suffering, but so are men, children, and Mother Earth. It has created an imbalance in the world and ourselves. It is overwhelming, even paralyzing, as it is essentially thousands of years of abuse of the feminine essence.

Feminine Energy and Empowerment

A historical and holistic perspective from Jeff Migdow, M.D.

When we look at the history of societies, we see two basic paradigms: cultures based on a belief in energy that connects our material existence with other levels of consciousness, and societies who only believe in the material plane.

Our current society and ancient Rome are good examples of materially based cultures, where what we experience with our five senses is reality, and everything else is a mental projection, or hallucination. Our materialistic culture believes that all our experience resides within the physical body, including our thoughts and feelings. The ego mind rules this way of thinking, and we are constantly in our mind, using experiences of the past to create the future.

Vitalistic, or spiritually based, cultures such as ancient India, China, and Japan, the Incas, almost all indigenous cultures, and even the nature-based cultures of western Europe believe that there are more realms of experience. The yogic culture of India believes we have five bodies, including physical, emotional, mental, intuitive, and pure energetic. The Chinese believe all life is filled with the spiritual energy, chi. The Japanese also believe in this energy and call it ki. The Native Americans refer to it as the Great Spirit, and the yogis call it prana.

These cultures believe that life is multidimensional and that it is permeated by universal, eternal, conscious energy—the basis of all life. These cultures also have an intimate connection with nature, who is known as the Divine Mother, Gaea, Pachamama, the Holy Grandmother. In these cultures, nature is the most powerful goddess, known as Mother Earth and considered as important as God, known as Father Sky. We may separate faces and forces but all is from one source, otherwise known as Creator/Great Spirit/Source/Divine/Universe. In vitalistic society, humans are naturally intimately connected to nature and the whole universe. We are ruled by our intuitive self, which is in direct contact with the present moment and guides us from our heart. There is a natural respect for all forms of life and the universal energy that fills all things.

This is a far cry from our learned experience of a disconnected, individualistic life cut off from nature. In fact, in our religious materialism we aren't even allowed to delve into the spiritual aspect until after we leave our body. If we dare to fully embrace the spiritual lifestyle of our choosing and live it boldly, we do so with the possibility of being called crazy. We work so many hours and spend so much of our money on getting by that there is no time or money left over to take a necessary break to visit other parts of the world. The dollar rules the day, and even something as potentially transformative and healing as sex is maligned, commodified, and controlled by those who stand to earn the most money from it.

The important point of all this is that most of us were raised in a society that reinforces feelings of materialism and isolation and discourages experiences that lead us to feel a deeper connection to Spirit, without and within. Most people I have known have had multiple experiences in which they feel a close connection to nature and Spirit, but the experiences are fleeting, and these people are not sure how to integrate these experiences into their practical life or even how to communicate these experiences and feelings to others.

The driving force of this materialistic society is masculine energy. In masculine modes of thought, black-and-white thinking and forceful action are prioritized while nuanced, intuitive feeling is minimized. Men naturally rise to the top in this system, as they tend to be more linear thinkers, and women learn to strengthen their masculine traits in order to survive. Remember that prior to the English popularization of pants a few centuries ago, women always wore flowing skirts and dresses. The skirt represented the circle of life. The circle of the skirt kept us connected to Mother Earth and her life-giving energy. Now, it's not just our thinking and action, but also our clothing that has driven us to a constricted way of thinking while our intuitive aspects have been shriveled. Even people that we look up to for their creativity—the singers, musicians, dancers, and artists—are controlled by their agents and the system, leading to drug use, depression, and suicide among them.

All of this is extremely disempowering, which is where our main problem lies. When the male aspect dominates the female and the ego mind takes over the intuitive power, we become slaves to our fickle, judging self. We become more concerned with how we look rather than how we feel, with our judgments of ourselves rather than our inner knowing. Thus our lives revolve around situations we cannot control. We lose the ability to have power over our lives or feelings. And as we feel more disempowered, we become more attached to how we are seen in the world and give up our power to our spouse, boss, doctor, and society. Once I choose to make my life revolve around what *your* mind thinks about me, I truly have lost my ability to have power over my life.

How do we break out of this way of life when it is all around us? When TV, billboards, radio, and even our peers encourage us to make more money so we can spend more money in an endless cycle of work, accumulation, stress, and tension? What's the point? The truth is, if materialism is the only reality, there isn't much point at all—thus the rampant depression, anxiety, insomnia, and physical stress in our culture.

Our saving grace and one true hope is that if we look at history, there have been millions of people who have been raised in spiritually oriented cultures. Even if you were raised in a materialistic culture, if you're reading this book, you know firsthand that there's much more to life than what we are taught. In fact, if we believe the yogis, Zen masters, medicine women, and shamans who have existed in all cultures as far back as we can document, then there are multiple dimensions of reality that we can experience, all the way to the Source. And it is all possible in this lifetime.

This shift toward the masculine appeared around 2,200 years ago as matriarchal, circular societies shifted to patriarchal, linear models. This corresponds to the beginning of the Piscean Age. It's also the time when the yogic scriptures were simplified from long epic stories, such as the Mahabharata, to logical chains of thinking in the Yoga Sutras of Patanjali and other works. Astrologically, we are now moving into the Aquarian Age, which represents the balance of male and female. Thus our feminine aspects are becoming stronger again, leading to an upswing of interest in yoga, tai chi, native rituals, ceremonies, and natural medicine. As this shift strengthens, more and more of us will feel our intuitive, connective, feeling aspects strengthen. This will set off a major shift in individual and collective consciousness, but not without lots of work.

In order for us to experience our deeper, truer selves and a pure connection to Mother Earth, Gaea, we must throw off the chains of our past actions and thinking by using tools such as those described in this book. These tools will allow us to go deep within, to acknowledge where we've blocked our intuition or creativity, where we've let ourselves and others down, forgive ourselves, and move on. As we go through this process, we begin to feel our power return. Then we will have the courage to dig deep inside to find the places where our fears and energy blocks lie, to go through the deep catharsis of letting go of all that keeps us from experiencing life fully. As we come through the other side, we find our full power and courage emerging, enabling us to live our lives in full presence and joy.

The Other Side of Power

As I see at Boot Camp for Goddesses time and time again, when we are reminded of the unfair treatment women have received over the course of history, we often no longer feel confused, guilty, or frustrated. We have clarity and hope for ourselves and our future. It is as if the chains of this internal anger are lifted, and we see what we are truly fighting against—an evolving cultural handicap.

The biggest gift we can give ourselves, our family, and the world around us is to channel our frustration and process our emotions so that we can take actions that are productive and self-affirming. When we accept that our emotions are part of being a woman and human, we can heal. Ask yourself the following questions:

- What part of me does not feel worthy of love, abundance, health, wealth, and success?

- What are the beliefs I have learned from my religion, family, and culture that keep me from being whole?

- What are the emotions, feelings, and experiences I have bottled up that stop me from living in my true nature and working to my true potential?

- When have I let the material, rational culture around me thwart my own dreams and goals?

- What can I do to act from the deepest, purest expression of my being?

Once you understand your answers to these questions, you can begin to see yourself as you truly are and start tapping into your goddess power.

When Native Americans weave a rug, they purposefully create an imperfection to remind them that nothing in life is perfect. They do it to remind us that if we are always looking for perfection, we miss where the magic and miracles in life happen. South American natives' ponchos are initially split in two parts—the left side represents the spiritual and the right side the physical. When they are then sewn together down the middle, they represent our ability to learn how to weave in and out of both worlds. Just as we learn how to use the opposing forces of spiritual and physical health, we must also learn how to weave in and out of them gracefully. The natives call this shapeshifting. We all have this ability if we are willing to tap in and use it. This sort of emotional intelligence is naturally infused in the world around us—we just have to know where to look for it. As I say to the women, if we cannot feel our deepest emotions, how can we call ourselves women—the intuitive, wise, emotional ones? When we use our emotions as energy—to heal, move, create, change, and be creative—we can accomplish everything.

Just as the healer or shaman works with all levels and frequencies of energy without fear or judgment, we must also learn this native intelligence in order to heal. As women, we naturally do this in everyday life, shifting nimbly between our many roles as mother, lover, professional, maiden, wild woman, and wise woman. We are blessed as women to have this gift of flexibility and flow. When we learn to tap into and access the deepest part of our emotions and put our intuition into effect, we unleash our Goddess/Warrior selves.

We have always had this power; we have just forgotten how to use it. We all know when one of our children is threatened, we channel our fear and anger from the bottom of our bellies and souls and prepare to fight to the death for our child. When this happens, you are calling on the Hindu goddess Kali, the goddess of destruction, the Amazon warrior and lioness. It can be scary to anyone who witnesses it and even to ourselves. Our anger is frightening, and yet when we learn to channel it properly it is the fire that sparks our spirit and soul to fight for justice and balance.

When we give birth to a child, we physically go through one of the most painful things in life, yet we are willing to go there for the outcome of that precious child. Men wonder how we do it. We bleed, push another being out of us, yet we are still alive in the end.

As women, we are multidimensional, as are all goddesses. When we can tap into the deepest part of our soul, we can call on these powers and gifts to guide us, heal us, and challenge us to be the powerful women we truly are. Yet most of us are becoming heavy and stagnant in our minds and hearts. We have lost this ancient gift and technique for fear of truly owning the totality of our power and beauty.

Ask yourself the question, "What does *feminine* mean to me?" Most people look at that word as being soft, compassionate, loving, sweet, pretty—all adjectives with no action behind them. These words are the handcuffs that keep us stuck in a system that does not allow us to be who we truly are: feminine, powerful, beautiful, free, wild, passionate, intuitive, nurturing, and self-loving.

To help you on the road of rediscovery, investigate the lives of the three generations of women in your family—your mother, grandmother, and great-grandmother. What are their maiden names, their stories, their gifts? In a patriarchal society where names are passed down by the father, women are denied knowledge of their lineage, which is a means of disempowerment. By exploring your matriarchal lineage, you add the power of your ancestors to your own as you unlock their secrets and let their gifts come to light. Only then can we restore the broken parts of ourselves and keep our wounds from being passed down to the next generation.

As women, our very purpose is to teach the power of this love. But in order to do so, we must be able to love ourselves—our *whole* selves, the physical, emotional, mental, and spiritual sides of our existence.

The following story was written by my niece, a goddess in training:

GODDESS STORY

All about a goddess girl, or what my aunt Sierra taught me:

A goddess girl cares about herself and other people. She sees God on the inside and outside. A goddess girl cares about her body, so she eats good food and exercises all the time to keep her body strong and healthy. She likes to play sports and be connected to nature. A goddess is comfortable and proud of being a girl and loves herself. A goddess also is graceful and strong. She loves animals and loves to talk about God and Spirit. She gives thanks by praying, singing songs, and performing rituals to Mother Nature and God. She loves to talk to Spirit, loves her life and the world's life too.

I love being a goddess!

—Gianna

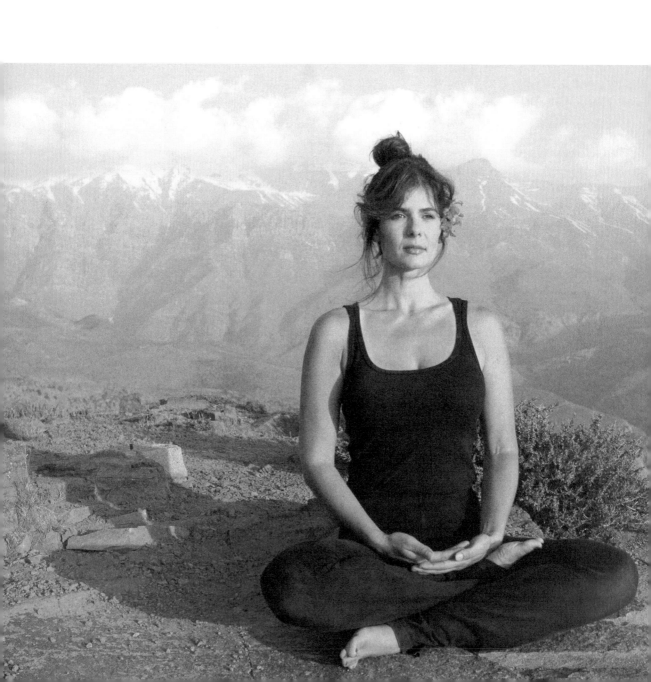

Chapter 2

THE SPIRITUAL BODY

When we want to get in shape, turn our life around, or start a new chapter, most of us think we need to start with the physical body. We think if we lose weight, get in shape, and fit into our skinny jeans, we will finally be happy and all our dreams will come true. But what I learned on my healing journey after my near-death experience is that revitalization doesn't work that way. It starts with the spiritual self and works its way out to the physical.

As I healed from my trauma of losing a child and nearly dying, I found myself wandering around totally numb. When I was technically dead, I felt supported and empowered by God. Here on earth, though, I felt lost and confused, because I no longer knew how to communicate with the people around me. They all knew I had been through a traumatic experience, but I could never find the words to explain what had happened to me. All I knew was I had to live a new life and move toward this newfound power—the power to surrender.

Out of this despair, I regained the power of prayer. I prayed every night, just as I had when I was a child having free-flowing conversations with God and nature. Now I told God that I knew what I had experienced on the other side was real, and I begged and pleaded to find this same feeling while I was alive: "May my eyes, ears, and heart be open to receive your information, and please have mercy on me." This was my way of asking the universe to bring it on, but to be gentle in the approach. If I could not experience that warm, abiding love here on earth, I told God I would rather die. I knew if I stayed where I was, without changing, it would become more painful to be alive than it would be to die.

The Other Side of Power

I had always thought that power came from being smart, beautiful, and in control of my own destiny and the destiny of others. And the natural accompaniment of this power, in my mind, was success—money in the bank, an impressive title. Now I began to see that this was only one definition of power. The loss of my child and my uterus gave me the gift of getting in touch with the *other side* of power—the ability to be receptive, observant, patient, nurturing, trusting, and abiding. I learned from this experience that true power didn't come from domination, but from surrender.

When I say surrender, I don't mean giving in, but rather giving up what is no longer of service to you. We are always looking for more—more power, more money, more stuff—but we are rarely willing to give up anything to make room for new developments. We think that giving up our unhealthy habits will be too painful or too much work. And we are scared to ask ourselves, "What is it that I truly desire, require, and deserve?" The problem is, if you do not know what you desire, how are you ever going to find it? And if your life is too full of other stuff, how will you ever make room for it?

I used to think it was better to always know what my next move was than to be still and silent so I could hear my own heart guiding me. I had thought that being still was being vulnerable, that stopping and listening was wasting time—that being still was being unproductive. I didn't realize it at the time, but I had been completely neglecting the feminine, spiritual aspects of myself.

Reclaiming the Feminine

Before I go any further with my story, what do the words *feminine* and *masculine* mean to you?

When I ask this question to men and women alike, I often hear definitions that are typical and judgmental. *Feminine* conjures images such as vulnerability and weakness. *Masculine* often elicits responses such as forceful, demanding, domineering, powerful, and selfish. The problem is, these ideas bring up a lot of pain and anger in both sexes.

We are conditioned to think masculine means "man" and feminine means "woman"— two separate identities, two separate energies. But in reality, masculine and feminine are flip sides of the same coin and continually influence each other—so much so that they eventually become one and the same. Everything in nature contains these two forces. The sun, with its direct, intense, expansive energy, is masculine; while the moon, which is cool, reflective, and mysterious, is feminine. We humans also contain both energies, no matter our gender, and our culture needs both the masculine and the feminine in equal amounts in order to survive.

In Native American tribes, men would not go to war unless the women told them to go. A woman's intuition and insight was greatly respected, for she knew how to talk to Spirit and see the future. Many women today still have this power, but they suppress it, because it is not rational, respected, or even safe to do so in our culture. Think of all the women who were called witches, killed, or thrown in the loony bin for their intuitive gifts. The peril is that by denying these gifts, we deny our true selves. It is no wonder that women in America today are more than twice as likely to be on antidepressants than men.[14]

When we do not respect and claim the energy of the masculine and feminine equally, we prevent ourselves from becoming whole, from healing and being of service to ourselves and to Spirit. We suffer because we are out of balance—in our lives, in our environment, even in our brains. When we favor one mode of being over the other, we create an imbalance in our hormones that can compromise our health and keep us from having the strength to make our dreams and visions come true.

To redefine power, we have to redefine the words *feminine* and *masculine* and understand that they don't oppose each other but rather complement and make each other whole. Here is a list of the characteristics of both energies. Can you see how one set of characteristics is appropriate sometimes, but not all the time?

14   See http://neuroskeptic.blogspot.com/2009/08/us-antidepressant-use-doubled-in-decade.html.

Feminine	Masculine
Receptive	Protective
Fluid	Linear
Intuitive	Decisive
Reflective	Expansive
Allowing	Forceful
Flexible	Unyielding
Observant	Focused
Compassionate	Rational
Persevering	Explosive
Patient	Driven
Devotion	Freedom
Peaceful	Fierce
Creativity	Manifestation
Stillness	Movement
Silence	Sound
Rest	Action
Intimacy	Self-reliance
Emotional	Intellectual
Graceful	Solid
Be	Do

Even a warrior has to have the right balance of male and female energies. She needs to be observant and still, so she will know when to take action and use force. A warrior who only possesses male characteristics is reactive, violent, forceful, and dangerous to herself and her community. The feminine side of power provides information and lends the insight to know when and how to tap into the masculine aspects of ourselves—taking action, following through, and moving forward. In order to manifest something, we must be creative and have an idea; in order to be focused, we must observe so we can decide where our focus should be; in order to take action, we must be still so we can know when to take action. *Everything in life starts with feminine energy first.*

A Single Step

When I knew I needed to leave my old life behind, I had no idea what I wanted to create in its place. My search for answers led me to a New Age shop, where I hoped to find something that would help me make sense of what I was feeling. A friend of mine owned the store and suggested I visit a place called Kripalu. When I heard it, I thought, "*krupah*-what?" She handed me a catalog of the yoga retreat center in the Berkshires, and as soon as I saw it, I knew it was the place. Being a personal trainer and in good physical condition, I thought, "How hard can yoga be? Touch your toes, breathe, relax, blah blah blah." I did not know why I was supposed to be there, but I knew inside this was the place.

Once at Kripalu, I did a month of yoga teacher training, a month of massage training, and several months of a spiritual lifestyle program. During this time, I cried—a lot. I had not expected that the process of learning how to go deeper would bring up more pain. At first, I thought to myself, "For God's sake, Sierra. Get off the floor. You are so much stronger than this. You do 100-pound squats and spend every day in the gym. What's wrong with you?" I felt like the Wicked Witch of the West, crying, "I'm melting, I'm melting!" What *was* melting was my ego as I dug deeper into my soul. But the more tears I shed, the more space I created in my mind and heart. I no longer fought to hold my feelings in. I gave up the old hurts and attitudes that no longer served my growth. And in doing so, I created space for what I desired, required, and deserved: peace, joy, and a new start instead of the constant pain I had become accustomed to. I learned a new definition of core strength—to stop running away from the pain and sit still long enough for it to rise and pass on its own. I walked every morning in the fields at Kripalu, where there is a beautiful bronze six-foot statue of Saint Francis. Every morning, I meditated and prayed next to it. I had found a new daily ritual. Nature was the only place I felt safe and connected. I could sit in silence to hear my own heartbeat and listen to the sounds of nature.

When I was done with yoga training, I learned so many tools to work with my mind, body, and emotions, yet there was something still missing. I knew there was more information for me to discover. I did not know where or how to find it, but I most certainly knew Spirit would guide me. One late summer night at Kripalu, I sat down under a tree with a couple of friends. I pulled out a large map of the United States, tied a bandana around my eyes, and asked my friends to move the map around so I would not know where all the states were. I held up my left hand and ran it slowly over the map. When my hand started to get hot, I placed it on the map and took off the bandana. I was pointing directly to the four corners of Utah, Colorado, Arizona, and New Mexico. I had made the decision to trust that Spirit would speak to me through my intuition, and now I had to be brave enough to follow it.

I awoke the next morning, headed back to New Jersey to get my car, my dog, and my one suitcase, and left for Four Corners. My yoga training had taught me about detachment, and now I took this all the way to the edge. I gave away my jewelry, clothes, and furnishings. My family did not know what to do with me. Their first thought was that I was crazy, but they respected my wishes by not stopping me.

When I arrived at Four Corners, I saw wild mustangs running free, slept under the stars, took baths in the rivers, and went on many hikes. I ended up living in New Mexico for five years and becoming friends with the Navajo, and then living another five years in Colorado, living off the land in tipis and a log cabin. I did many ceremonies with the Native Americans, and I found a friend and teacher in Mother Earth. I learned how to work with the elements and how to trust that everything I needed would be provided. And it was. At the start of my journey, I had no plans and only a little bit of money. Yet throughout, people gave me food, money, and clothes. I met many people from many places, and I was living the dream of being totally free.

On my travels, I talked to many Native Americans who taught me their ways, such as the sweat lodge ceremony, which represents going into the womb of Mother Earth in order to be reborn. I found these rituals and ceremonies to be the missing piece I was searching for, because they provided a connection to Mother Earth—the most powerful goddess of all. I loved the action behind their prayers and rituals and the ways they prepared their mind, body, and spirit to be of service to Spirit. They believe the only thing we can give back to Spirit is our sweat and tears. There is nothing on this planet that Mother Earth has not provided for us. The only way we can give back is to keep our bodies and our hearts clean and clear so that when we kneel down on Mother Earth and under Father Sky, we are humble.

I have never in my life felt more whole and spiritual. It was if I knew these ways and beliefs already, and I was rediscovering a lost part of my soul. The songs, the language, and the ways were easy for me to learn. I had no fear, only respect and devotion to the teachings. When I told them about my near-death experience, they understood. They didn't think I was crazy; they knew I had been rebirthed and blessed by Spirit. And to think we have all but destroyed such a beautiful culture and way of life for fear of dealing with the unknown and the wild part of our nature—our innate native wisdom.

While I was in New Mexico, I visited the Kundalini Center to practice with Yogi Bhajan and learn about tantra and kundalini yoga. I loved the teachings and learning more about Goddess, and then my spirit led me to Santa Fe. I had faith I was always heading in the right direction, and I was always rewarded with a sign that I was. When we truly listen, Spirit speaks to us in many ways—through animals, signs, and people. I arrived in Santa Fe late at night to witness a holy city that felt like the most beautiful place on earth. I stood in the middle of the plaza, looking at a historical church with the moon and millions of stars shining on it as if God were saying, "Look at me." At that moment, I saw a familiar face—a statue of Saint Francis. I was on Saint Francis Drive, looking up at the Saint Francis Cathedral. I could not believe my eyes. I never looked outside of myself again for the answers.

Contacting Your Intuition

As Rosalyn Carter once said, "A leader takes people where they want to go. A great leader takes people where they don't necessarily want to go, but ought to be." Spirit is a great leader, and your intuition is the way Spirit speaks to you. Follow it, and it will take you where *you* need to be.

How many times have you known who was on the phone without looking at the caller ID? How many times have you sensed or dreamt your child was in danger or needed something? How many times have you *not* listened to this inner voice and wound up embroiled in a situation that drained your energy? Let's say when you first met a man, some part of you said *something is not right* and pleaded with you to walk in the other direction. But you are so conditioned to look for the knight in shining armor instead of reality that you decide to shut this voice up. You say to yourself, "He is not so bad. I can change him. He has great potential." And five years later, you find yourself in a big breakup, perhaps even a divorce and a custody battle, all because you turned off your intuition.

Here's another example: you love eating pizza from the place that makes it with the fresh mozzarella and the great sauce. One day, your intuition tells you, "Do not eat this today," but you eat it anyway—and it triggers a whopper of an allergic reaction, or a migraine, or a massive case of eczema. Choices like this happen again and again and again because we are taught to deny our intuition. Because if we *were* to listen to it, we would be free of all attachments and realize we have the power to protect and provide for ourselves. Each of us has the power to make our dreams come true, yet we choose to give it away or shut it down. We choose to settle out of fear: fear of being alone, fear of failure, fear of not providing for our children. When we learn to listen to our intuition, we hear our higher self, which always knows exactly what we need to do to move closer to our true selves.

Goddess of the Spiritual Body:
PACHAMAMA

Pachamama, also known as Gaea, also known as Mother Earth; Mother Earth has many names. She also has many faces, depending on where you live and what your spiritual practice is. We humans are all her children. She sustains, nurtures, and holds us unconditionally. Mother Earth and Father Sky are our true parents, meaning that our birth parents here on earth are just as human as you are and are the means but not always the way. And when we are able to tap into this nurturing relationship with

Descriptors
FOR THIS GODDESS

Healing, whole, holy

Mother Earth and the abundance of Father Sky, we can heal, bringing wholeness and a feeling of holiness back into our lives.

Message from This Goddess[15]

I sing a song of love from the stones of my body, from the high peaks of my mountains, from the hot sands of my deserts. I caress you with green leaves, green plants, and green grasses. I feed you from my breast, the earth. I soothe you with sparkling rivers and refresh you in my ocean. My song of love is my body, the earth. It is there to feed you, clothe you, and house you. Learn my song, and it will heal you. Sing my song, and it will make you whole. Dance with me, and you'll be holy.

How Pachamama Works in Your Life

Do you remember when you were a little girl and loved to be in nature, playing with other children or your animals and climbing trees? Do you remember making mud pies, going to summer camp, or spending your vacations at the lake, on the beach, or in the woods? Our parents had a reason for letting us play outside all day: to get us out of their hair, yes, but also to allow us to be wild and free.

Do you also remember when you stopped climbing trees? Do you remember how you had to learn to take up less space and not be so wild by crossing your legs, sitting up straight, and sitting still—not to go inward, but so you would look like a lady? Didn't that piss you off sometimes? Of course, there is a time and place for everything, and of course we need to have manners, but why is it acceptable for boys to act childish and play rough—as evidenced by the old saying, "Boys will be boys"—while girls are always expected to "know better"? It's as if our elders were telling us, "Get used to bad behavior from men, honey, because you will live with it the rest of your life," when it would be so much more helpful to hear, "It's okay, honey. Boys are just born that way and they cannot help themselves. That is why God made girls, because they are so much wiser and know better." We women have a different kind of wildness. It's not about being rowdy and untamed, however. Our wildness is fierce, yet our natural understanding of the magic and mysteries of life is something boys have a harder time understanding.

---

15   Used with permission from Amy Sophia Marashinsky's *The Goddess Oracle* (U.S. Games Systems, 2006).

As children, all the time we spent outside helped keep our life force strong, vital, wild, and free. Yet we didn't know that's why we longed to get outdoors—it was just natural, and it felt great. Today's children have lost this right, and we are responsible because we have taught our children to fear being alone in nature—after all, they could be raped or kidnapped. And then we require them to sit all day in school behind a computer, and we wonder why we are having so many problems in our culture today. The most powerful healing tool for challenged kids is to get them in nature. And they love it, because it helps them act on the innate intelligence that every human being is born with.

All of Mother Nature's elements provide vital pieces to our health and happiness: fire keeps our spirit strong and alive, wind cleanses our negative thoughts and our aura, water cleanses our toxins and soothes our emotions, and the ground holds, warms, and heals us. Spending time among the four elements unites our four bodies. Yet when was the last time you encountered any of the elements, much less all of them, on a daily basis?

South American and North American native cultures believe the human race has umbilical cords that connect them to Mother Earth. They believe she is our true mother who loves us unconditionally, yet they also know that her elements are the strongest forces on this planet, capable of completely kicking our ass—as she is doing now. Mother Earth is telling us, "Wake up! You have abused me and used me enough. You have thrown off my balance, and now we all suffer. You humans have to remember that I can survive without you, but you, my dear children, cannot survive without me." It's the same way my own mother used to joke when I really made her mad: "Honey, I brought you into this world; do not forget that I can easily take you out of it."

Because they believe that they are permanently connected to Mother Earth, there is no fear of death in the native cultures. For thousands of years, they have buried their dead in a fetal position, knowing that the departed would be reborn in one form or another. They were made of Mother Earth, and they will be born from her again. This type of knowing is not an intelligence we learn in school. It is a wisdom that has been passed down for thousands and thousands of years. As we looked at earlier, symbols of Mother Earth date back 30,000 years—her arms are always open to Father Sky, her breasts are bountiful, and her belly is fertile. She is depicted giving birth to her children: the plant, animal, and mineral kingdoms, and even art in all its forms—music, painting, dancing, weaving, and more.

I found my true mother, Pachamama (as the South Americans call her), when I lived off the land in the Southwest. That's where I truly realized that no other human being would ever be able to fulfill all my needs, but Mother Earth could. When I had this realization, I felt it in every one of my bones and cells. I felt aligned with my inborn intelligence again, and it healed me and helped me become whole and holy again. I learned to forgive on a whole other level. I let go of past pains with my own mother and father. I learned how to nurture myself, claim my own space, and embrace, embody, and own my wild woman nature—the mystery and magic of my spirit and soul.

I have had decades of education through the school system, the church, yoga trainings, massage school, healing schools, and more. Yet none of them taught me the importance of connecting to Mother Earth. How come? Because the feminine essence of Spirit has been taken out of healing as a whole. We think as long as we have intellectual knowledge—if we go to school, if we study—we will know everything we need to know. But that is learning from the outside in. It is not nearly as powerful as learning from the inside out. When we learn from experiencing our emotions, intimacy, reflection, and creating a connection to Spirit, we truly understand how something works and how it connects to everything else.

What Is the Spiritual Body?
HONOR YOUR TRUE NATURE

The spiritual body is ruled by the fire element and the spirit of Mother Earth. It is the divine spark, the light within. It is our sense of self, the center of who we are. It is the undeniable knowledge that we are creatures of God.

The spirit is an intangible, nondimensional body that provides us an abundance of energy and wisdom to know, feel, and sense that we are a part of something larger than ourselves. Think of it as our *truest* nature—otherwise known as the higher self, the god within, the divine, Spirit, universal energy, the higher power, and consciousness. The spiritual body connects the spiritual self with the human self, and it consists of eight muscles that help it stay fit, lean, flexible, balanced, clean, and focused: higher self, energy, life force, filter, intuition, consciousness, connector, and unconditional love. Rebuilding the spiritual body establishes a solid, abiding sense of self.

Muscles of the Spiritual Body

Higher Self

The higher self is an integral and intimate aspect of ourselves that remains aware of our fragmented aspects and our wholeness simultaneously.

The only time we feel true satisfaction is when we fully experience love and Spirit for ourselves. Connecting with the higher self takes practice, refinement, dedication, and discipline. You will receive from this practice what you put into it. It is important to understand that there are no beings, planes, or dimensions *outside* of ourselves. All beings, planes, and dimensions of consciousness exist equally right here and now, within and around us.

Your higher self naturally wants to help you evolve to be able to access the many higher frequencies that exist in the universe: nature, Spirit, spirit guides, and true love.

Your higher self is spontaneous, creative, open-hearted, fearless, indomitable, patient, accepting, and spiritually connected. Your higher self is speaking to you when you embody feelings of rootedness and power:

- I am real.

- I am satisfied.

- I surrender.

- I am free.

- I commit.

- I love.

Energy

Energy is an infinite source. Energy is manifested through frequencies, vibrations, sensations, feelings, and emotions with *action* behind them. Frequency is how fast or slow energy moves. Vibration is the feeling that is given off from energy. Sensation provides awareness of energy's presence. Feelings bring forth internal awareness, and emotions are the responses we have to feelings.

Considering how vigorous this muscle is, it's not surprising that energy is what motivates or distracts us from being whole. Energy motivates us physically, moves us emotionally, intrigues us mentally, and heals us physically. The most powerful energy, of course, is love. Love is not only an emotion but also an energy with action behind it. As we'll see over the course of this book, unconditional love is a cross-over energy that we store in all four bodies as a memory, reminding us we are always whole and always worthy.

Not surprisingly, the spiritual body is the first body to recognize love. It takes action by serving as the vehicle that transports the energy love provides to the other bodies. In fact, it is the spiritual body's job to keep this energy flowing constantly so that it moves within us and radiates from inside us. It's the spiritual body's job to keep love alive.

How does this happen? Believe it or not, it happens the same way we keep the physical body alive—with food. The only difference is that the *spiritual body* requires *spiritual food*.

Spiritual food is made up of the experiences that strengthen our sense of self—those events and occurrences that remind us we are creatures of God and that God lives within us. Spiritual food comes in those moments when we are overwhelmed by the truth that love is an internal and external expression of God. It is when this love is present that we can honor the god within us and glimpse our spirit's purpose.

What happens when love doesn't flow within us? What happens when this energy doesn't move outward? What happens when it becomes stagnant? Sadly, pain and suffering manifests in all four bodies, and it usually starts with the spiritual body. This pain and suffering slows down the energy, vibration, and frequency of the spiritual body, weakening its ability to ward off unhealthy forces. These negative forces eventually affect the other bodies because the spiritual body, having been weighed down, loses its strength to protect the other bodies, thus creating discomfort. We might even think of this discomfort as the first manifestation of disease, appearing in the spiritual body as an early warning signal. Disease, illness, and sickness come from a lack of energy balance in our body and soul. The spiritual body, our most sensitive body, is the first body to register this lack of balance.

Balance of energy comes from a healthy respect for the opposing forces present within each individual—such as yin and yang, male and female, outward and inward—that unite to keep our energy moving. When these opposing forces unite and create balance, we feel the result as our life force.

Life Force

Male/female, love/hate, yin/yang—these are polarities that have their own energies, intelligence, and wisdom. They are stored within us and surround us. Think of what happens when you take a positive and negative charge of a battery and unite them—they ignite, creating sparks, energy, and power. Our life force works the same way. Life force is created when opposing forces are sparked together to create movement, power, and growth. This life force powers the spiritual body, and the spiritual body filters the life force to the other bodies to create balance.

Filter

Another job of the spiritual body is to act as a filter. It cleanses and protects us from unwanted, unhealthy energies that constantly surround us. These unhealthy energies drain us of our own personal energy and life force, leading to an imbalance within us, and therefore leading to an imbalance around us.

Unhealthy thoughts, overloaded emotions, negative people, and an unpleasant physical environment—these are just a few of the unhealthy energies that can weaken the spiritual body, leaving the other three bodies vulnerable and open to harm. The spiritual body shields us from these unhealthy energies so they cannot penetrate the other bodies. It detects the presence of these energies by trusting, listening to, and following the spiritual body's most powerful tool, intuition.

Intuition

Intuition is the bridge that connects our spiritual body to the other three bodies. Intuition is the part of ourselves that is receptive to information that comes in through the heart and mind. It is the capacity to feel with our minds and listen with our hearts. It is an internal message revealed to us through our sixth sense, that inner voice we all talk about but sometimes fail to hear.

Through our intuition, we have the ability to sense, feel, or see that something is right or wrong; we can tell when something is off balance or in balance. It's what many people refer to as a "gut feeling."

It is also through intuition that the energies feeding the spiritual body are revealed. These energies are both known and unknown to us. Our intuition is the bridge to see, feel, and touch upon the unknown mysteries of God's creations—universal energy, Mother Earth, angels, the spirits of people who have died, galaxies, solar systems, and other mysteries that the human mind can't even begin to grasp. We communicate with these energies by using our intuition. Think of it as sonar, tuning in to the energy surrounding us and the energy inside us; these subtle messages protect us and give us the vital information we need to stay whole. They are messages from the god within us, sent to help and guide us to the people, places, things, and experiences that we are meant to discover.

To locate your intuition, you must stop, look, listen, be present in the moment, and feel everything. When we listen to and trust our intuition, our next step is revealed. Instead of guessing and wasting time, trusting our intuition keeps the spiritual body in alignment with our higher purpose. Using and trusting our intuition strengthens the spiritual body and our relationship with ourselves, others, and, of course, the god within. When we follow our intuition, we access wisdom and intelligence of the known and unknown, leading us to conscious choices made equally with our mind and our heart.

Consciousness

The spiritual body helps us maintain the purest and clearest state of our heart and mind. When we allow the ego and personality to hear, receive, and trust the intelligence of our intuition, we no longer separate ourselves from this intelligence—we *become* it. It's in this connected space that we can recognize the god within us and experience true consciousness. When we are experiencing consciousness, we are filled with faith, hope, and belief in a higher power and our own purpose. Consciousness is existence in its most lucid, serene state.

Connector

The spiritual body is our connector to life force, higher self, energy, love, intuition, and consciousness. All of these resources bring us inward to see, feel, and sense the god within us. And, when connected, we can see God surrounding us. We may know this intellectually, but experiencing it is radically different. We can only experience the god within us and surrounding us by connecting to our:

INTUITION: When we stop, listen, and feel what is within us as well as around us.

ENERGY: As we feel the flow of love within and allow love to radiate out.

LIFE FORCE: By maintaining a balance of the opposing forces that live within us.

CONSCIOUSNESS: When we hold the purest, clearest state of mind and heart.

The spiritual body acts as a connector by infusing consciousness into our human heart, the home of our emotions; our spiritual heart, which knows the purpose of our life; and the heart of our soul, which knows we are creations of God. These components of our heart exist as one whole, but are also individual depths we must search. When these three elements of our heart work in balance, they become one, and we are truly conscious. The spiritual body connects this consciousness not only to our heart, but also to the three other bodies.

Unconditional Love

Unconditional love is the inherent knowledge that resides within each of us that we are all one, and that all of God's creatures are made of the same elements and have the same intelligence and wisdom within them. Unfortunately, modern cultures tend not to teach how we can connect with and tap into these resources in order to draw energy from them and ultimately use them as a source of healing power.

A Healthy Spiritual Body

To tap into the spiritual body's resources, we must understand that finding balance within is necessary for our growth and happiness as human and spiritual beings. The spiritual body is the first body to maintain this balance and pass it on to the other bodies. This balance is a conscious memory within us, reminding us of our true nature, and it is our responsibility to preserve and sustain that. We can maintain this balance by using and trusting our intuition to guide us to conscious choices that are healthy choices. But to do this, we have to first let go of the busyness in our minds. We need to take the time to be quiet so we can hear our inner voice. This practice strengthens our intuition, senses, and instincts—therefore strengthening the spiritual body. When we hear our inner voice, we can ask questions and receive answers. We begin to trust and follow our gut feelings and believe in both the known and the unknown forces available to us.

Qualities
OF A HEALTHY SPIRITUAL BODY

Intention, intuition, integrity, honesty, faith, hope, belief, trust, abundance, receptivity, meditation, prayer, joy, bliss, compassion, unconditional love, nonjudgment, self-love

If we don't listen to our intuition and take the answers we receive seriously, the spirits of the known and unknown will not take us seriously, and our spiritual body will suffer from lack of nourishment, which is also a lack of balance. When we practice using our intuition, we understand who we are, why we are here, and what our purpose is—we glimpse the interconnectedness of life. With this clarity comes spiritual gifts that help us move forward toward our dreams and visions. Our life has direction and meaning; we feel energized and alive. There is a constant flow of life force and energy. We can tap into any resource we need to help us, heal us, or energize us, because the spiritual body is conscious and open to receive what it needs—and equally open to discard what it does not need.

A healthy spiritual body senses the discomfort of unbalanced, unhealthy energy; it can determine which energies are not of service and discard them. A healthy spiritual body has a strong sense of integrity—a centered self with personal boundaries. A healthy and strong spiritual body builds a foundation of integrated strength, balancing the physical power of force with the intuitive power of wisdom.

An Unhealthy Spiritual Body

When the spiritual body loses its balance, it will have difficulty recognizing love. When the spiritual body becomes underweight, it isn't able to fight the unhealthy energies that can bring further harm to the other bodies. This happens when the muscles of the spiritual body that once kept it healthy and functioning—such as intuition, energy, and consciousness—deteriorate from lack of use. And the other bodies are affected too. The mental body, for example, becomes unable to focus or concentrate; the emotional body overreacts; and the physical body becomes sluggish, causing our metabolism to slow down. We no longer radiate from within because we are starving from spiritual malnutrition.

When the energy that once kept the four bodies connected to one another doesn't work and becomes heavy and stagnant, this weight creates fatigue, stress, and hypersensitivity. Our thinking becomes irrational and our hearts numb. We become snared in an analytical search for answers to our existence and lose trust in a higher power. It is a slippery slope; the spiritual body will descend into a constant state of confusion. Doubt and an overload of distracting information will rule the day.

As you might imagine, an unhealthy spiritual body creates enormous amounts of stress. Stress is far and away the worst enemy of the spiritual body, because stress leads to unhealthy unconscious thoughts, feelings, and actions. If conscious thought leads to healthy choices, then we know where unconscious thought will lead us. We start to feel we are losing control of ourselves and our environment. Our reason for existence is no longer about motivation but about manipulation. Our thinking originates from a place of fear, scarcity, and the desperation of sheer survival. Greed, jealousy, and anger poison the heart, mind, and spirit. Suffering from spiritual emptiness, this void of self-awareness makes healing an impossibility. We can no longer spread our wings to fly; how could we when the spirit is so wounded it has lost its *faith* to fly?

Qualities OF AN UNHEALTHY SPIRITUAL BODY

Disharmony, irritability, loneliness, lack of trust, fear, unforgivingness, blame, victimization, lying, lack of faith and hope, lethargy, lost sense of self, loathing, judgmental, lack of self-love and unconditional love

In such dire straits, we start asking the big questions: Who am I? Why am I here? What is my purpose? Why is this happening to me? The heart and mind battle to find balance and consciousness. Somewhere in our journey we have lost our ability to simply believe in a higher power that is there to help us.

Each one of us has seen or experienced situations that can create an unhealthy spiritual body. Consider these all-too-common examples:

THE MIDLIFE CRISIS: The disturbed mind, heart, and ego searching for meaning, justice, and purpose.

THE REALITY OF DEATH: We fear the reality that we are indeed destructible, mortal, and our lives will eventually end—oftentimes this highlights a fear or a lack of love in our lives.

MENOPAUSE: A disorienting but natural cleansing process of the mind, heart, body, and emotions that women must go through to return to their sense of balance with their creativity, voice, wisdom, and strength.

DIVORCE: The separation and loss of a lasting and loving intention.

ILLNESS: A disease or traumatic experience that forces us to stop and reevaluate our lives.

ADDICTION AND ABUSE: A lost sense of self.

These experiences are all wake-up calls for us to return to our four bodies, to feel our four bodies, and to fight for our own self-worth.

An UNHEALTHY SPIRITUAL BODY

A medical perspective from Jeff Migdow, M.D.

IMBALANCES IN THE spiritual body—ruled by the fire element—have deep, far-reaching effects. When we are cut off from our spiritual self, we experience a disconnection from the fire of life itself: energy. This leads to lack of faith and hope, feelings of separation and aloneness, and a loss of connection with our intuition.

In my work, I find that this will manifest as either lack of fire in the system or the fire having no stability and moving throughout the person, leading to emotional depression, deep mental anxiety about life itself, insomnia, chronic fatigue, and the development of addictions such as overeating, alcoholism, drug use, Internet abuse, and other behaviors designed to numb us to this deep spiritual despair. These behaviors then lead to secondary physical diseases such as obesity, high blood pressure, diabetes, fatigue, and acid reflux, as well as the social problems of breakdown of communication in relationships, sexual acting out, and physical and emotional abuse.

A study done in the 1980s showed that even though India was steeped in poverty, compared to the average American, the incidence of depression, anxiety, alcoholism, drug use, and other diseases was much higher in America. This study found that the main difference was that the average Indian felt a deep connection to Spirit and God, an intrinsic connection to the universe that was manifest in various activities during the day, while the average American felt a disconnection from Spirit and God.

Disease of the Spiritual Body: A Case Study

In the late 1980s, I saw a middle-aged, affluent man who was suffering from depression, insomnia, and high blood pressure. He initially saw me for the blood pressure, but within fifteen minutes it was obvious that his main imbalance was on the spiritual level. He was extremely wealthy, but he had lost two million dollars in the stock market crash. He still had millions of dollars in assets, but his faith had been broken. Even with his affluence, he felt depressed and couldn't sleep due to constant worry; he was sure he would lose all he had. It took a few sessions to get to the point where he could admit that stress wasn't his main problem; rather, it was lack of hope and disconnection with Spirit.

He was actually a rich man in many ways, not just financially—he had a loving wife and children, good friends, and the potential to work for decades to come. He had become so tied into experiencing who he was by how much profit he made that the monetary loss made him feel two inches tall. Through the tools I taught him to reconnect with his spirit self—including affirmations, prayer, and gratitude for what he loved in his life—he was able to reconnect to gratitude for what he still had on many levels, and he began to believe again that he was intrinsically supported by the universe. His mood improved, his sleep deepened, and his blood pressure eventually went back to normal. Our last visit was six months after he had first seen me. Although he had lost more money, he felt healthy and whole and had begun to enjoy his life again.

This case shows the importance of staying connected to the spirit within us, as this enables us to withstand the ups and downs of life in a much healthier, smoother way.

SELF-TEST TO DISCOVER THE CURRENT STATE OF YOUR SPIRITUAL BODY

The following questionnaire is designed to enable you to find your strengths and weaknesses in the spiritual body. It is also beneficial for strengthening self-awareness, which is key in being able to objectively see yourself clearly and from there be able to create more openness, strength, and balance in your life.

Take time for each question, and answer in a way that feels truthful to you. If you have areas where you feel like you aren't being honest, know that these are the places in which you tend to fool yourself. Usually these are the areas that need the most work.

Give yourself 5 points for *always*, 4 for *often*, 3 for *sometimes*, 2 for *occasionally*, and 1 for *never*. Then add up your totals for each body to get the grand total. This will help you objectively see where you stand in this body. As you move through this book and take the tests for the other bodies, compare the totals to see where your imbalances lie. We suggest you do each of these questionnaires every one to two months to check your progress and give you time to reflect.

Questions **Key**: always (5 points), often (4), sometimes (3), occasionally (2), never (1)	
1. I feel a spiritual presence during my day.	
2. I find time to meditate every day.	
3. Prayer and deep reflection are tools I use when I am confused or unable to find a clear path.	
4. I am aware when I am disconnected from Spirit.	
5. My intuition speaks to me when I need direction.	

6. I use visual tools such as prayer beads, spiritual artifacts, beautiful art, and tarot or oracle cards to help center and open to my inner knowing.	
7. I use deep, restorative breathing to help energize and revitalize myself.	
8. I can feel when my spiritual body wants to give me information.	

Tally your score by adding up the points that correspond to each of your answers, and jot it down in a notebook or journal. Although 40 is a perfect score, where you fall on the scale today is not as important as seeing your scores improve over time, both numerically and in relation to your other bodies. (You don't want one score to be off the charts, with others far behind, for example.) As you test all four bodies, you'll begin to see how you can bring more balance to your entire being. If, for example, you scored a 36 on your spiritual body test, and later realize that your physical body fitness is only a 14, you can use that information to bring those numbers onto a more equal plane, perhaps by meditating less and working out more.

Strengthening the Spiritual Body

Although we may not understand why we are going through pain and suffering at the time, sometimes purpose can be seen from a distance. It's very possible to grow from suffering. By taking the time to examine our most painful experiences, we can begin to recognize what is off balance within us and ultimately add to the intelligence of all four bodies.

Rebuilding the spiritual body establishes an even stronger sense of self. For the spiritual body to be whole and balanced, all eight muscles we discussed earlier—higher self, intuition, consciousness, unconditional love, energy, life force, filter, and connector—must be nourished and nurtured in all areas. No area in the spiritual body is insignificant.

AN INSIDE-OUT WORKOUT FOR
THE SPIRITUAL BODY

When people talk about a workout, they usually mean something that involves a gym, a trainer, a treadmill, free weights, a yoga class, and so on. My inside-out workout, however, is a little different. It's exercise for all four bodies, and the goal is to create suppleness, flexibility, balance, focus, and full range of motion in each body. In doing so, we can rehabilitate, recycle, reprogram, and reenergize *all* of our bodies.

All of the following tools and exercises are rituals to nourish and feed the spiritual body, strengthening the spark of Spirit within. I call it spiritual food that feeds all eight muscles of the spiritual body.

Ritual and Ceremony

A ritual is a set of actions often thought to have symbolic value performed within a certain context, whether it be religious, cultural, or familial. The word *ritual* may bring up judgment for many; still today, when I say this word in my workshops, women admit it makes them think of witchcraft or something bad that they should not participate in. But once they realize the true meaning, they are released from the fear. What does this word bring up in you?

When you see how many rituals we have in our daily lives, we can then let go of the fear of this word. Brushing your teeth, going to the same yoga class every day, and eating pizza every Friday night are all rituals—a set of actions that have a symbolic value to you, such as going to yoga class to be in shape, eating dinner with the same people each week to enjoy friends and family, and brushing your teeth to be healthy and clean. Even common actions like hand-shaking and saying hello are rituals. We are literally surrounded by rituals, and the world would be a far less caring place without them.

A ritual can be an action that you do daily, seasonally, or even only once. Examples include holiday family gatherings; celebrations for the full moon, new moon, equinoxes, and solstices; funerals; and baby showers. These are all rituals to celebrate the cycle of birth, death, and rebirth. A ritual of this nature also can be done once in a lifetime to mark an important rite of passage, such as childbirth, menarche, marriage, and death. Initiation ceremonies such as baptism, confirmation, and bar or bat mitzvahs are important rite-of-passage rituals.

A ritual can also be an act of connecting with Spirit. Examples of this type of ritual include meditating, praying, lighting a candle, participating in sweat lodge ceremony, and honoring the Sabbath. These rituals fulfill emotional, spiritual, and physical needs. They strengthen our inner core and higher self, and create social bonds with others, leaving us feeling whole and holy, with a feeling of being connected to Spirit and to others.

Many native cultures have customary rituals and ceremonies that help them stay in alignment with Spirit and Mother Earth. These rituals are a practice of discipline, commitment, and perseverance, and some are quite challenging, such as the vision quest, sun dance ceremony, pow wow, and sweat lodge. They are often done yearly. Smaller, daily rituals are also performed—such as making an offering to Mother Earth each morning to show thanks and appreciation for all she provides. A daily ritual can also be a song, a prayer, or an act of kindness. Regardless of the scope, making ritual a regular part of your life takes commitment, intention, time, and a sincere desire to be of service to Spirit.

What rituals do you have in your life, and how do they make you feel connected to Spirit and yourself? It could be the sun salutations you do each day to honor and give thanks to the sun, or the candle lighting you do every Friday night to mark the beginning of the Sabbath.

My everyday ritual is to sage myself (see below for more information about burning sage), set my intention for the day, and ask for guidance from and give thanks to Mother Earth and Father Sky. I also give an offering to Mother Earth and her animals by singing a song on my morning walk and leaving a gift of food, such as cucumber peels, carrots, lettuce leaves, or pieces of fruit—whatever I feel I have that will give back to her and her creatures. I do this ritual with my nieces.

Every morning in the shower, I awaken with a cold rinse and pound on my body to bring blood flow to all the organs and glands. I make loose fists with my hands and tap my lower back, thighs, buttocks, feet, head, neck—every part of my body. It is great for circulation and brings on life force full force. To be clean and fresh for the day, I also visualize the water cleansing my mind, thoughts, and energetic body as the water swirls down the drain. It is as if every cell turns on the light bulb.

Here are some ideas for small rituals you can incorporate into your daily life as a means of staying connected to Spirit.

- Leave any food that you do not eat, such as the peels of your cucumbers or carrots, out in your yard, perhaps under a favorite tree, as an offering to Mother Earth to say thanks for the food she provides. Even if you live in a city, leave bread for the birds on a windowsill. Children love this exercise; it teaches them the value of give and take, balance, and respect for nature as a whole. They will ask for it every day and help keep you disciplined in your daily rituals as you also build family fun and connection. As you get ready for dinner, ask your child to peel the cucumber, cut the carrots, and make a bowl of goodies for their offering. It also builds the discipline of saying thanks—for you and for your children. How many times have you taken from Mother Earth and not given back, too busy to stop for minute and do a prayer of thanks? And how do you feel when your children take from you and don't acknowledge the time and energy you've spent by just saying thank you? This exercise helps remedy both situations.

- On your next hike, leave an offering of appreciation and gratitude for all that Mother Earth has given us. We forget her elements are alive; the fire, wind, water, and earth spirits that give us life, hold us and sustain us, provide all we need to have a healthy, vibrant body and life. Yet we so easily forget how to give thanks on a daily basis. The least we can do is leave her a gift of gratitude such as a crystal, a flower, or a prayer; or hug a tree and offer your thanks to Mother Earth. You could sing a song, recite a poem, or chant a mantra—whatever calls to you. Wait to see how she responds to you.

Benefits of Ritual

- Creates an opportunity for Spirit to speak to you.

- Teaches you how to give thanks and creates time and space for you to do it every day.

- Cleanses your energy and helps you leave the past behind and start each day with a fresh mind, heart, and spirit.

- Balance of give and take.

Thank mother earth

Soul Searching (Tratak)

During Boot Camp for Goddesses, I am always amazed at how excited women get once they are finished with this next exercise. At first they are petrified, because we rarely look into someone else's eyes in our culture—it is seen as invasive or impolite. But what this exercises teaches is that the eyes truly are the window to the soul, and when we gaze into others' eyes and allow them to gaze into ours, we let our own light shine and we receive information from Spirit.

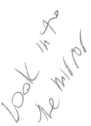

look in a
the mirror

This exercise shows you how powerful your intuition is, and it does it in a very practical way that you can use as one of your most powerful tools in negotiating your daily life. Wondering if he's the guy for you? Want to know how your loved ones really feel? All you have to do is look into their eyes.

This exercise can be done alone or with a partner. It strengthens your concentration and promotes stillness of the mind and heart. Known as *tratak* in ancient India, this practice enables you to see and access the reflection of Spirit in your own soul or another's. It is a very intimate and deep exercise whether you do it with yourself or someone else.

Do it for anywhere between one and fifteen minutes—aim to work up to at least seven minutes to have a full experience. It's a very deep healing practice if you choose to be strong enough to truly look within.

When you look into the mirror, do you only see your external self? Do you judge yourself and say, "I am not beautiful"? We have become so conditioned to think beauty is only external, but true beauty is not only to be seen, but also felt. This exercise will help you see and feel your true inner beauty—the kind that radiates from within.

To do this exercise alone, sit or stand in front of a mirror and stare into your eyes with a soft gaze. It will be hard to focus at first and difficult to concentrate on both eyes. You will be drawn to one eye, then the other. Breathe into your heart and continually check in on your breath. Be open and receptive to anything that pops into your head, and try not to judge. The deeper you look into your eyes, the more information your higher self will reveal. Of course, fear or a rational thought may come in to distract you—just continue to concentrate on your breath and your eyes.

You may start to see, sense, and feel things; this is all normal. You may even see yourself change from one form to another; you may go so deep that you glimpse a past life and see yourself wearing a headdress. Do not judge or fear the information you receive, just accept it.

You may also see that one eye looks totally different than the other—perhaps the left eye is half-closed and sad, and the right eye is bright, like a laser beam. The right eye is the eye of the ego—it reflects our personality and the different masks we wear. The left eye is the eye of the soul. The right eye is protective, hard, and judgmental, engaging the fight-or-flight response, while the left is receptive, loving, and soft. Our goal as humans is to have our personality and our soul be in harmony with each other. When they are not in balance, it will show in our eyes and our energy.

Perhaps you'll see colors around your head, which is your aura—your own energetic field. Regardless of what exactly you see, your energy will continue to shift and flow as you continue. You may be amazed by how your energy is warm and healing one moment and protective and scared the next. As you look deeper into your eyes, you are going deeper into your own soul, and it can be either exciting or frightening. Whatever happens, just stay with it, and whatever you're seeing and feeling will soon shift into something else. Each person and each experience is different.

It takes patience and practice to be open and receptive. This exercise requires a discipline of the mind and heart. Do not get frustrated at first if you cannot do it—it's a very normal reaction. But keep at it. You will love this exercise once you master it.

Soul Searching with a Partner

To do soul searching with a partner, sit in a comfortable cross-legged position facing each other. Each of you should place your left hand, palm up, and right hand, palm down, then place your hands so that your hands are on top of each other, palm to palm. Sit with your spine tall so that you have room to breathe deeply. Stay silent as you gaze into each other's eyes for at least seven minutes. Once the seven minutes are up, you can each share your experience.

This exercise is very intimate and can feel confrontational or uncomfortable at first—just breathe without judgment. You will have a hard time looking into both eyes simultaneously, and your focus may go in and out like the lens of a camera. Trust your intuition to guide you. Do not lose focus. You are just there to be open and receptive to any information that is trying to come through.

The moment judgment comes in, breathe into your heart. The moment your mind wants to make sense of it all, breathe in. Do not allow the rational mind and ego to steer you away. You may see things, such as colors or shapes, or feel things, such as sadness or joy. Take in the information as data, not judgment. You may see the person one moment as an old, wise medicine woman and the next as a child running through the fields. Do not think you are crazy; you are just taking in information. You or your partner may not be able to see anything, and that is okay, too. Remember: no judgment. Like any other exercise, it takes practice, patience, and discipline. You may feel uncomfortable and resistant to sharing this exercise, or your partner may not be able to look into your eyes. It is just the energy at the present moment, and energy always shifts into something else, like the flipping of a coin.

GODDESS STORY

After a soul-searching exercise during a Boot Camp for Goddesses, one of the goddesses spoke up to the group to share her experience. She said she kept seeing these beautiful white clouds in her partner's blue eyes. She was mesmerized by her partner's peacefulness, yet she felt sadness at the same time. The partner, hearing this information, started crying. At first, the woman was also upset, thinking she had upset her partner. Then her partner revealed that her father had recently died and had told her, "Honey, anytime you need me, just look at the clouds and know I am always watching over you." Both women cried and realized that Spirit was with them both at that moment.

The intuitive mind can see beyond the obvious, into the mystery and magic of the universe. This exercise shows us that Spirit is talking to us all the time, but our rational mind doesn't listen or trust the information that's coming through. There are so many of these beautiful stories. It helps women see that they are made of the same stuff—Spirit and Love. It helps women feel close to one another, get over their intimacy issues, and bring their competition with other women to an end. They see Goddess in each other and in themselves.

The Goal:

You will know you have mastered this exercise when you are open and receptive to intuition without needing any outside validation. You make an inner decision based on the information you received.

*O*ne attendee was commuting back and forth to the campus where Boot Camp for Goddesses was being held. When we started the first night of the retreat with a sharing circle, she was surprised and disappointed—she thought we would be doing a hard-core physical workout. She told me that she was considering dropping out of the retreat because it was not what she expected. I asked her to stay one full day before she made her decision to leave. Some women want to leave right away because they realize there will be contact with others and they came for an external workout, not an internal one. This woman did return the next day when we did the soul searching. She decided to go home and do the soul searching with her husband that night. The next day, she told us what had happened, and she had everyone in tears.

They did the exercise for fifteen minutes, then they shared their experiences with each other. When it came time for her husband to share, he was in tears. He said, "We have been married for eighteen years, yet I have never felt so loved and connected to you before. I can truly see you and know why I love you."

When returning home from Boot Camp for Goddesses, a mother of two young boys, ages eight and ten, came home to them fighting. She immediately sat them down, taught them the soul searching exercise, and reconnected the love of the two brothers again. They then discussed their feelings and put it behind them—a great tool for children to learn!

Altar

In Hebrew, an altar means "a place of slaughter or sacrifice." You can see why some people have a bad reaction to this word. An altar is used in many spiritual practices and religions, including Buddhism, Hinduism, Catholicism, Judaism, Wicca, Paganism, and others. In all these traditions, an altar is a place of prayer, sacrifice, and offering—*sacrifice* meaning giving something of yourself to Spirit, whether it be your intention, prayers, sins, or a gift.

Every woman needs an altar, whether it be in her house, office, or even her car. I have one in all three places. In my car, I have a small crystal, a bottle of essential oil to keep me calm and focused, and an angel pin on my dashboard to watch over me. In my office, I have an altar with a candle, a goddess statue that represents my work, a dollar bill with lots of zeros added to feed myself and my business, a quote I love about leadership and success, and tokens of all the places I have traveled to with my work to help keep me focused and abundant. In my house—my most sacred space—my altar is where I meditate and pray. This altar is in my bedroom, on my dresser. On it is my sage, sacred feathers, crystals, water, and incense. They are all placed on a beautiful scarf made by women in the Amazon jungle—a holy place I visit yearly. This reminds me of how much I know and do not know; how much I have grown and how far I have to go; how these women and all women around the world are connected like the weaving of a spider web.

Each morning I am home, as soon as I wake up I sage myself, say my prayer, and sage my entire house. The smell of the sage helps clear my mind and my house of yesterday's energy so I can start a new day. I set my intention, then allow the magic and mystery of the universe to show me the way. And I am always amazed that when I take the time to get still and be silent, information from Spirit comes when I least expect it. This one ritual has taught me to visualize what I desire, require, and deserve—to visualize it and then let go of striving and allow Spirit to bring it to me. The biggest challenge always is to be careful for what you wish for; ask yourself if you are truly ready for it and if you feel worthy to receive it.

An altar is a place where a woman can refocus, regroup, honor, and ignite her fire of passion and compassion, and put herself into alignment with her goddess self. It is her sacred space where she is safe to stop, look, listen, and feel what is going on within and around her. Her altar is a place of devotion where she can come and have her most intimate conversations with God, her higher self, and even her guides.

You can make an altar anywhere in the house, but keep in mind it is your sacred space—not everyone else's to touch and play with. Just as your body and energy are sacred and not to be squandered or polluted, so is your altar.

Here is an example of how others can steal or invade our sacred space. Once your children or partner sees your altar, they will want to touch your things. You can help them to understand by setting boundaries and explaining that it is your space, with your personal objects that you do not want disturbed. They will listen, but nine out of ten times they will not follow your instructions and they will touch the altar anyway. They are merely acting out of excitement, but it is possible to be disrespectful without being conscious of it, and it also shows how they will disrespect the altar of your personal space and the temple of your body. But if you help them create an altar of their own, you can use it to teach them boundaries: if they take something off of your altar, you can take something off of theirs and not give it back until they have earned it. It will help them understand the consequences of their choices and behavior in a subtle and loving way.

Making an altar for your children is a wonderful way to teach them how to cultivate the discipline to practice being silent and still so that they can connect with Spirit themselves. You must remember that stillness and silence are learned activities. Next time your child does something wrong, do not silence them and send to the corner; this only teaches that silence is bad. Instead, send them to their altar and ask them to reflect and look inward. Help them find an offering, such as a flower, poem, song, or stone, to leave on their altar and make it an enjoyable experience. When they do not feel safe or are having a hard time, they can come and sit in front of their altar and speak to God, their friend. They can hold a crystal or a rock they found on their hike—whatever makes them feel powerful, calm, and connected—and learn how to be still and have faith.

The Goddess Altar

Find a cloth or scarf you like and a clear, flat surface somewhere private, quiet, and safe. It could be a table or dresser, a big windowsill, or it could be outside in your garden. Lay your scarf on top of the surface, and then place your sacred objects on top of the scarf. Your objects can be anything that makes you feel connected to Spirit. Try to use things that reflect all four elements—water, fire, air, and earth. Use a candle to represent how you are igniting the fire within. Have incense, sage, or an essential oil to represent air, a small bowl of water with sea salt for the water element, and a crystal, stone, or dirt for the earth element. Then make a small ritual for yourself of lighting the candle (to represent your spiritual self and the fire element), burning the incense or sage (for your mental body and air), dipping your fingers in the water (emotional self and water), and holding the crystal or rock (for the physical body and the earth), and do it every day as a means of connecting with the god and goddess within.

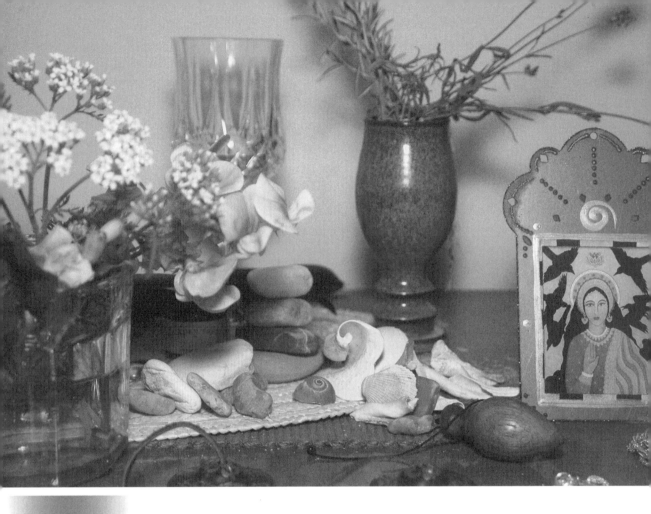

An example of a goddess altar. There are four elements that should be represented: fire (candle), air (sage or incense), water (a bowl or vase of flowers), and earth (rocks, crystals, shells, etc.). In addition, have photos of places you have visited (or would like to visit); loved ones to pray for; and statues or photos of goddesses to remind you of your true feminine power and essence. Above all, choose objects that help you connect to your spirit.

If you have heard scary stories of witchcraft and sacrifice, the word *ritual* may bring fear for you. If you notice this happening during your own ritual, breathe into it and know that you are only honoring the Spirit within. Know that now is the time to change this belief and that you are working to make a new version of history—or, in this case, *her*story.

It is good to change the objects on your altar seasonally or whenever the mood strikes, since changing the objects will change the energy, and energy is always changing and flowing.

Meditation

We have 50,000 thoughts a day, with the negative far outweighing the positive. The practice of meditating creates space between our thoughts so we can hear our own inner voice. By quieting the mind, you create space for your intuition to come through much more clearly. Different techniques have evolved all over the world to help us experience Spirit directly by focusing the mind on the breath, a part of the body, a concept, or a sound, and then becoming so present with the point of focus that all other thoughts quiet and the intuition can finally be heard.

Meditation is the practice of stillness and silence. It is a way to connect to oneself. Being still and silent is internally taking action.

Stillness and silence are learned activities. When we take the time to be quiet, we hear our inner voice. We can then ask ourselves questions and filter out negative thoughts and emotions. Meditation can help us find answers and understand who we are, why we are here, and where we are going.

Beginning Your Meditation Practice

Sitting is the best position for meditating (see photo, page 38). It allows you to practice stillness and silence by giving you a comfortable position in which you can stop, feel, and listen.

The most important part of meditating is making sure you are comfortable and the spine is straight. This opens the diaphragm and heart, allowing the breath to come into the heart and fill the lungs, which end at the top of your shoulders. You can sit in a chair, lean against a tree, sit with both legs crossed Indian-style or in the traditional yoga postures of full lotus or half lotus. You can even lie on the floor if sitting just isn't comfortable, with your heart facing up toward the sky or ceiling, palms open, and toes turned out.

As you sit, allow your thoughts and feelings to rise to the surface. Do not title them good or bad, just allow the sensations of these thoughts to arise, and let them go by breathing into them. By doing this action, you are allowing yourself to let go of what is no longer healthy so that you can hear your inner voice more clearly. It is like weeding out the old thoughts, belief systems, and demons so new seeds and thoughts can grow. This also allows your intuition to come through so that it may steer you, instead of allowing your doubts, fears, and insecurities to lead you in the wrong direction and waste your energy and time, like a mouse on a wheel.

When you have mastered meditating, your mind no longer feels like it is in a maze; rather, your thoughts become like a labyrinth: you can always see the center—the point of your existence and your purpose for being here—which then allows the heart and mind to work as one.

- If you have a hard time sitting still, it's okay. The more you meditate, the better you get. You are building a new muscle.

- Light a candle as an expression of your intention to honor yourself.

- Sit up straight, opening your heart and spine.

- Stare at the candle flame for one minute. Set a clock so that you can sit without taking your focus off the flame. Count how many negative thoughts you have in a minute.

- Sense and feel how many times you want to move away from being still and silent and how many distractions you had in one minute that took your focus off the flame.

Other Ways to Meditate

- On a hike or walk, sit under a tree for a couple of minutes, your spine straight, and just listen and feel the beauty of nature. Take in the view and creatures that surround you. Nature automatically slows your heart rate, cleanses your personal space, and gives you a calm, peaceful feeling that slows down the mind.

- Close the door to your office, sit in your desk chair, and remain in silence and stillness for 5–15 minutes; see if you can feel your breath moving into your heart. Close your eyes and focus on your breath, placing your attention and intention on bringing forth awareness into those areas of your body where your breath cannot reach. Breathe in and out of your nostrils only, which will slow the heart rate and bring in a peaceful feeling to the mind and body. Breathe into every cell; visualize tension subsiding with every exhale. As you breathe in, visualize white light expanding into every cell and cleansing away toxins, tension, and unhealthy thoughts. When exhaling, visualize the color gray flowing out as you let go of what is no longer needed.

Advanced Meditation

More advanced practices include taking a long walk in meditative silence, having a day of silence, or even, as indigenous cultures do, practicing a vision quest—a four-day inner quest, fasting while you search for direction, purpose, and how you can be of best service to Spirit. Other forms of detoxification are also very helpful for the spiritual body. Although intense, during these rituals you are in such a state of clarity, your body and mind become a vehicle for Spirit to come through and guide you on your journey. You receive visions and experience the mystery and magic of life. In similar Eastern practices, yogis do a seven- or ten-day retreat of silence.

Benefits:

In meditation, we start to realize in this deep state of reflection how much energy and time we waste in talking and projecting our life force. Meditating on all levels is a great discipline to go inward and face the demons of the ego, the lower self, and understand how these things keep us from connecting to the true source of our existence.

Practicing meditation leads to physical relaxation, emotional calm, mental clarity, and spiritual opening. Thousands of studies have been done all over the world during the past eighty years on the physiological effects of meditation. Herbert Benson from Harvard proved in the 1970s that not only does meditation create a deeper spiritual connection, but it also has many physical benefits, such as relaxation of muscles, lowering of high blood pressure, and decreased adrenaline release due to diminishing the fight-or-flight response. These studies led to his book *The Relaxation Response*.

Studies have shown that meditation shifts brain waves from the hectic beta waves our brain creates during the day to deal with stress to balanced alpha rhythm, which occurs when adrenaline, the fight-or-flight hormone, is diminished, and then into theta rhythm, which are extremely slow brain waves that the central nervous system creates when we reach deep stages of relaxation. With theta rhythm, endorphins are released in the brain, which lead to feelings of deep physical relaxation, mental peace, emotional joy, and spiritual opening. The more time we spend in meditation, the calmer the central nervous system becomes, the slower the brain waves get, and the more space there is to feel our spiritual connection. The result is a greater flow of energy and clearer, stronger intuition. The deep physical relaxation also helps normalize blood pressure, decrease heart rate, deepen our breathing, increase blood flow to the digestive system, and relax muscles and tendons, leading to diminished pain in common ailments like headaches, backaches, and arthritic pain.

Prayer

Every religion and spiritual practice prays. It is a way to communicate and have a relationship with the god within, the source of our existence. Prayer is also a way of giving back to Spirit, because we are validating its existence as our own. When we pray for and give thanks for all that we have and need to make our lives more abundant with health, wealth, and success, we are asking the universe to help us be the best that we can be for the greater good. And just like getting up in the morning and brushing your teeth, prayer is a way to cleanse your heart and mind of the debris the outside world projects on us all.

Prayer is the bridge that connects our human heart to the pulsating heartbeat of the universe. Singing, mantras, and affirmations are all forms of prayer that keep us in touch with the god within. Prayer invokes Spirit through words and rhythm. They can be spoken, chanted, thought, or sung, with or without the help of musical instruments such as drums. All of these techniques bring out the sound vibration of the words, which are designed to connect directly to Spirit. Prayer can be done alone or in a group.

Tools of Prayer

SONG: Singing a meaningful song connects your heart to the heart of the universe. An example of a song we sing in boot camp is: "Mother, I feel you under my feet. Mother, I hear your heart beat."

MANTRA: Repeating a word or words silently or out loud gives off a primordial sound that reflects the vibration of all the energy in the universe.

My daily mantra and the one I teach in boot camp is very simple. I sing this song to myself during my daily hike or yoga practice, or whenever I need a boost:

> *I am the twenty-first-century goddess.*
> *I am feminine.*
> *I am sensual.*
> *I am sexual.*
> *I am powerful.*
> *Don't ever mistake my kindness for weakness.*
> *And don't ever take me for granted.*

Tibetan Buddhists believe that repeating the mantra *Om Mani Padme Hum* out loud or silently to oneself cultivates compassion. In the kundalini practice, the following mantra is repeated:

> *Adi Shakti, Adi Shakti, Adi Shakti, Namo Namo,*
> *Sarab Shakti, Sarab Shakti, Sarab Shakti, Namo Namo,*
> *Prithum Bhagawati, Prithum Bhagawati,*
> *Prithum Bhagawati, Namo Namo, Kundalini,*
> *Mata Shakti, Mata Shakti, Namo, Namo.*

This mantra tunes in to the frequency of the Divine Mother—a primal, protective, generating energy. Chanting it eliminates fears and fullfils desires. *Adi Shakti* means the "primal power," *Sarab Shakti* means "all power," and *Prithum Bhagawati* means "which creates through God."

Kundalini yogis also chant:

> *Akal, Maha Kal*

This mantra means "Undying, great death." It is a powerful, life-giving chant that removes fear and relaxes the mind. Or, you could choose a mantra as simple as *Sat Nam*, which means "truth."

Or you could repeat the sounds of the chakras three times:

Lam—Root chakra
Vam—Sexual chakra
Ram—Solar plexus/stomach
Yam—Heart
Hum—Throat
Om—Third eye
Ommmmm—Crown

AFFIRMATION: An affirmation is a quote or prayer that keeps your heart and mind on track with your higher self and your connection to Spirit within. Repeating an affirmation allows your higher self to surrender to and trust Spirit, so you may let go of any negative thoughts, doubts, and fears that steer you away from the god within, creating pain and suffering. Some example affirmations are:

May my eyes, ears, and heart be open to receive you, Spirit.
May I know my truth.
May I see my truth.
May I speak my truth.
May I feel my truth.
Give me the strength, perseverance, and courage to follow my path.
How can I best be of service to Spirit today?

Or a shorter one:

No one and no thing will disturb my peace of mind.

How to Pray

Incorporating prayer into your life is an easy task. When you feel stressed or out of control, surrender those fears, doubts, or negative thoughts by singing a song that makes you feel connected to your heart and to the god within, or read a prayer or affirmation if you feel your mind is wandering toward the negative, and always give thanks and express gratitude at the end of the day for what you have. Never forget that things can always be worse; be grateful for the lessons you have learned, and be open to the new ones you will conquer with the help of God, Spirit, and the universe.

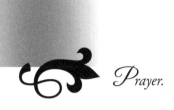 *Prayer.*

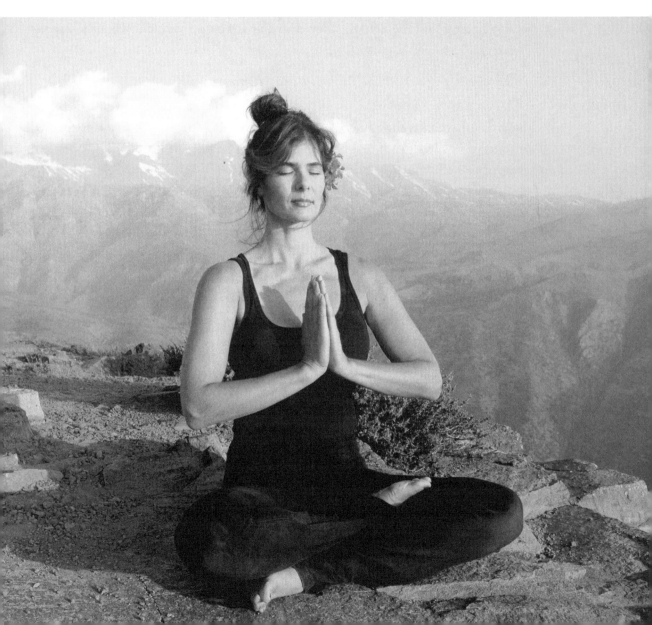

In yoga, sun salutations are physical prayers performed to honor the sun and the new day. To bring your sun salutations to the level of prayer, face east to greet and give thanks to the sun for another day.

Indigenous cultures have used prayer for healing the sick, fighting off an enemy, and asking Spirit for guidance. To hear the voice of Spirit speaking back to you is to experience the magic of the universe. It's an unexplainable but tangible gift we have all experienced at one time or another.

You can pray anywhere, at any time—in the car when picking up the kids, driving to work, stuck in traffic, in an uncomfortable situation when you need help, before bed, or anytime you feel the need to connect to Spirit, whether it be for help or to express joy or gratitude.

Uniting the Spiritual and Mental Bodies Through Prayer

Prayer can be a form of meditation. Rather than focusing on the breath, create an intention that serves the higher good and then verbalize or think it in a very focused manner. It involves the mental body in the spiritual experience. The more present and focused you are with the intention, the more powerful the vibration created in the spiritual body, the body of pure vibration. The vibration then leads to a shift in energy, which can then at some point manifest on the physical plane. We want to create only uplifting prayers, as these are for the good of all and release us from karma and tension. If you create a destructive prayer, then you are responsible for the results.

To try a praying meditation, sit or lie in a place where you feel safe and comfortable. Focus on your breathing long enough to enter a clear, focused state, then allow the prayer to emerge from within. It may be in your language or a mantra or a Native American chant—whatever helps you feel more focused and in touch with the spiritual body. Repeat the prayer aloud or in your thoughts, and feel it build in intensity and energy. Your intuition will tell you when you can let go of the repetition. Then sit in quietness, and let the vibration build in your spiritual body until you feel it moving out into the universe.

Benefits:

Prayer leads to an emotional calmness and feeling of support and safety. The experience of safety decreases the fight-or-flight hormones, such as adrenaline and cortisol, leading to the same feelings of emotional joy, mental calmness, and physical relaxation as meditation. These feelings and benefits are increased when we pray in a group or through chanting or song.

The rhythm of the chanting or singing of prayer is practiced by cultures all over the world, from Hindu mantras, to African drumming and chanting, to Christian, Judaic, and Islamic chanting of the Old and New Testaments in Hebrew and Latin. These rhythms deepen the heartfelt feeling of the prayer and increase the deep opening to Spirit. When prayer is chanted or sung, the deep vibrations lead to physical purification, emotional clearing and release, mental focus, and direct spiritual connection.

Smudging

For millennia, various herbs have been used for purification purposes. Many Native Americans believe that sage was the first plant that Mother Earth created. They dry the leaves and burn them to heal, purify, and bestow blessings on themselves and others. Native Americans believe that smoke is a representative of Spirit (since fire is the element associated with the spirit world), and that by bathing themselves in the smoke of burning sage, they could cleanse their spirits. It's similar to the use of burning incense in the Catholic tradition.

Uses for Sage

- Burn loose sage leaves in a wooden or metal bowl, or light a bundle of dried leaves (known as smudge sticks) and bathe yourself by fanning the smoke with a feather or your hand over your body.
- Purify the energy of your home or car with the smoke.
- Place sage leaves under your pillow to attract love and intimacy.
- Crush in your hands, rub together, and smell to get in touch with your inner wisdom.
- Use in stuffing for any wild game.

Where to Buy Sage

- Health-food, herbal, New Age, or whole-food stores.

 *Use feathers for saging.*

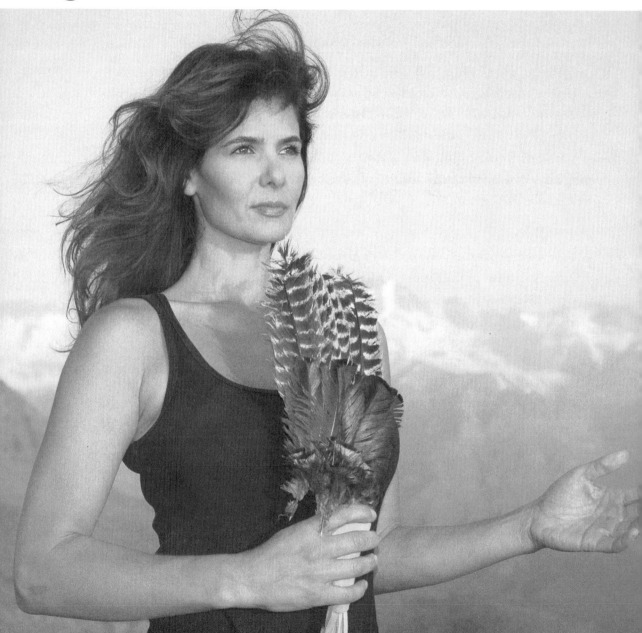

When to Use Sage

- First thing in the morning to cleanse your mind, energy, and space to get you prepared for the day.

- To cleanse your home, office, or car of any toxins in the air and to circulate stale air and energy, burn a smudge stick and fan the smoke into every corner.

- If you had a tough day, a conflict, or a gathering, cleanse others' energy by burning a smudge stick in your space. The smoke from the sage will cleanse and move stagnant energy.

- Healers use sage to cleanse and neutralize the healing space before the next client comes into the space.

Benefits:

The smoke of the herb sage has been used by cultures all over the world for spiritual purification. It is believed to release heavy, dark, dull energy from our energy bodies, allowing more light, clarity, and truth to come out. People who can see auras report that during a saging ceremony, areas of darkness or fogginess around a person weaken and sometime dissolve completely.

Animal or Angel Cards

We can use the insight of the ages by simply drawing a card from a deck; these cards may be groups of animals, angels, goddesses, or flowers. Everything in nature and on the spiritual plane has a specific meaning that relates to humans. For example, spiders and their webs represent connecting the energies of the bodies; ants, industriousness; bears, introspection. Each goddess and angel in history has a certain attribute. When we meditate and then pick a card, we draw the card with a special meaning to us. By meditating on the meaning of the card, insight, understanding, and intuition come to us directly.

These spirit cards are tangible objects that can validate exactly what we are thinking and feeling in the present moment, connect us to Spirit, and guide us in the direction we need to go. Whether we have lost our way because our mind is clinging to old belief systems and negative thinking, or our emotions are backed up and creating a fear of letting go, or our diet or environment is causing harm to our bodies, our energy and our intuition can get clouded. The cards steer us toward the unseen parts of ourselves and give us an avenue to hear our body's natural intelligence and wisdom.

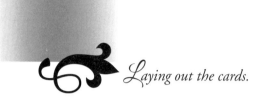

Laying out the cards.

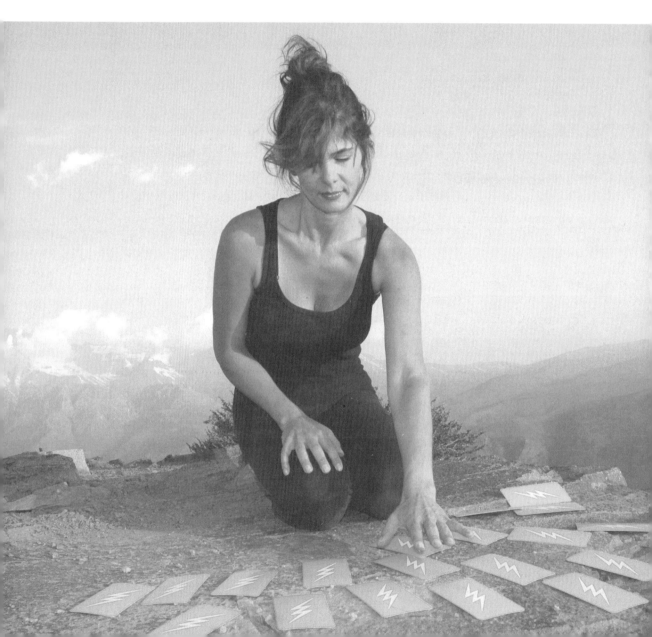

Wisdom Cards

There are many different types of card decks available in any bookstore, New Age emporium, or even gift shops and yoga studios. Choose one that calls to you, even if you aren't exactly sure why.

Your cards may come with specific instructions, but here are two simple methods that will work with any deck:

1) Shuffle the cards, and while you are shuffling, think of a very clear question you would like to ask. The clearer the question, the more precise the answer. Examples: *What is the best way for me to handle the situation I am in with my husband? What is the main point I need to express in the business meeting?* After thinking of your question, pick a card that you feel drawn to and read the explanation. The card you pick is not a coincidence—it is your higher self, guiding you to be the best you can be. Cards are a great way to grow, learn, love, and evolve at your own pace. By asking for an answer, you are surrendering to Spirit to help you, and the card you choose is a reflection of what Spirit is guiding you toward. Following through with this guidance is your responsibility; it shows your respect for Spirit when you follow the information you received. By not following through, you lose credibility with Spirit and become like the boy who cried wolf. If you don't trust and heed the information you received, the next time you need help, it may not be so readily accessible.

2) Place all cards on the floor or a table and spread them out so they are not touching each other. You can fan them out or make an arc like a rainbow. You want to be able to sense and feel every card in front of you. Play some meditative music, light a candle, and honor the spirit within who is awakening to guide and help you. Think about the issue or issues you wish to explore. Take your left hand—it represents the receptive part of ourselves—and hold it flat as you pass it two inches above the cards. Keep your eyes closed and feel all the cards as you ask your question. You may feel tingling, heat, muscle twitches, or sensations like electricity that steer you toward the card. When you flip it over and read about the card you choose, it is Spirit guiding you. It may not always be what you want to hear, but it is an invitation to awaken and open to the spirit within.

Once you've selected a card, meditate on what you have learned, and pray for guidance. A lot of times, we are confused by the clutter in our mind and heart. The mind will not allow what the heart wants to feel, and this exercise is a wonderful tool to find our wants, needs, and desires so we can walk on our path with clarity, purpose, hope, and faith, to know there is something helping us.

GODDESS STORY

My first evening at boot camp, Sierra laid out a deck of Goddess cards and explained how to hold your hand out to "feel" your card. But I felt instantly which card was mine—I did not need to use my hand. My eyes were immediately drawn to a card. I felt calm and did not need to hurry to make sure I got my card—I knew it was already mine. Funnily enough, as each woman went up to choose her own Goddess card, a couple hesitated with their hands over my card, but then moved on.

When I finally got up to choose my card, I saw that I had drawn Baba Yaga, the Wild Woman. The description of her was as if someone who really knew me wrote it about *me.* I've lived my life as a wild woman and have been chastised for my ways. Only my girls and my husband allow me this level of freedom and do not try to stifle this power. I felt I *finally* had a tangible description of who I really am and what my core strengths are. It was as if I had been given permission to do what I was put here to do, and I don't need to hide it or disguise it anymore.—*Elaine*

Benefits:

The benefits of drawing cards are the same as for meditation or prayer. By focusing our concentration on the picture and meaning of the card, we can go into a meditative experience, connecting to the essence of the card and drawing on deep intuition. This experience of intuition leads to feelings of support, safety, and clarity. Sometimes people go into a spontaneous prayer to the image on the card and feel great spiritual strength and hope.

This is also a great exercise for depression, ADD, and other focus-related diseases and illnesses. After practicing for a period of time, you will start to trust yourself, and you will pick up on creeping doubts and fears and not allow them to manifest in your mind or heart and lead you away from the god within.

BREATHING FOR THE SPIRITUAL BODY

Fire/Energizing Breath
SANSKRIT NAME: KAPALABHATI

Fire breath is the element of fire, energy, and force.

1. Come into a seated or standing position with your spine erect.

2. Place your feet hip-width apart and bend your knees slightly.

3. Make a triangle with your fingers and place it around your belly button, your index fingers pointing down (see page 20 for photo).

4. Inhale and allow your belly to expand.

5. Exhale forcefully through your nostrils only and pull the belly button in toward your spine, contracting the abdomen muscles. Allow the inhalation to naturally happen.

6. Repeat this movement twenty to thirty times and gradually pick up your pace. Work up to three to five sets of fifty. Keep tissues nearby.

Benefits:

When the belly button pushes in toward the spine, a surge of fire energy is released from the nostrils, creating heat to warm and massage your internal organs and the muscles of the heart and body. This heat stimulates digestion and elimination, which increases nutrient absorption and detoxification. Increased absorption helps rejuvenate and revitalize our cells, and the toxic release from the bowels helps us feel lighter and healthier, as our cells hold fewer toxic chemicals. It also releases and strengthens the diaphragm muscle, thus enabling longer and deeper breathing. The deeper breathing allows more oxygen to be absorbed, which energizes and revitalizes the cells, and increased carbon dioxide to be exhaled, which relaxes the nervous system and muscles.

This powerful breath also increases mental clarity by stimulating the flow of the cerebral spinal fluid that surrounds the brain and spinal cord, actually massaging and stimulating the brain cells. The stimulation of the brain cells and increase of breath and fire leads to an increased ability to focus the mind and boost vitality. With this clarity and vitality, intuition comes through much more easily. Jeff always does Kapalabhati before meditating or prayer. He finds it allows him to drop into a spiritual space much more easily.

Other benefits:

· Speeds metabolism.

· Strengthens the entire nervous system.

Precautions and Contraindications:

· Do not do if you are pregnant or menstruating; if you have high blood pressure, heart disease, an active ulcer, a hernia, or a lung condition; or if you have recently had a stroke or abdominal or thoracic surgery.

YOGA POSES FOR THE SPIRITUAL BODY

Yoga is the science and practice of self: self-awareness, self-acceptance, and self-love. Each posture will reflect your weaknesses and strengths. Are you able to go into pain or do you run from pain? Breathe, have patience, and know that yoga is not about being flexible but being in the present moment so that you can stop, look, listen, and feel what is going on within. It is about intention, not perfection. The physical body will always benefit from what you do internally first and work its way out to the external.

Lotus
SANSKRIT NAME: PADMASANA

The lotus is a floating water lily: the flower of light, beauty, and grace. Like a lotus, your tailbone and spine are the root and stem that keep your flowering body connected and still.

Your head is the flower of consciousness in bloom. The graceful lotus is not easily within reach—it takes perseverance and desire to touch it. Do you want to hold this graceful flower? The lotus of intuition unfolds as the true self.

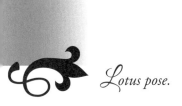 *Lotus pose.*

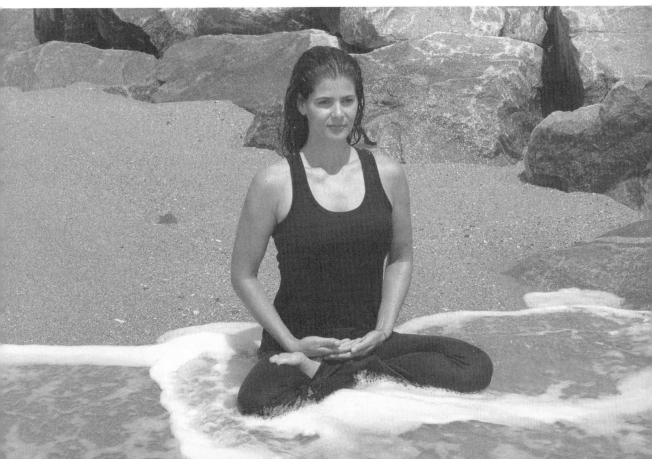

Entry and Holding Posture

Carefully enter lotus in stages, making sure your hips are appropriately open at each stage.

1. Begin in a seated position with your right leg crossed in front of your left.

2. Check that both thighs rest comfortably on the floor. If this is uncomfortable, try sitting on a pillow or place supports under your knees. The top of your pelvis should be higher than your knees.

3. When comfortable in this seated, cross-legged position, move to seated triangle by bringing the left lower leg out parallel in front of the body. Place the ankle of your right leg on top of your left knee and your right knee down toward your left ankle. (You can open your hips by gently pressing your thighs down and holding for five seconds.)

4. Once comfortable, press your pelvic floor down into earth, press the base of your thighs into the earth, and sense energy moving out from the hip joints through your knees.

5. Bring your right ankle up and rest it on the left thigh with your heel touching the hip joint. Turn the sole of your foot up and lengthen through the ankle joint. This is half lotus position.

6. Once you are comfortable, come into full lotus by bringing the left foot up onto the right thigh, with the left heel toward the right hip joint and the sole turned up.

7. Press both ankles down into the thighs and press the thighs and the base of the body into the earth as you lengthen energetically along the front and back of the spine and lift through the crown.

8. Rest the backs of your hands on the knees, palms open.

9. Allow yourself to relax and connect with the energy. Close your eyes and focus on the point between the eyebrows to center yourself in deep stillness. Attune deeply to deepen your inner peace and know the essence of your true self.

10. Repeat with opposite leg on top.

Lotus or half lotus is a stable posture to keep the spine straight and heart open to meditate. Hold one to three minutes for beginners. With each breath, breathe through the nostrils only. Hold for fifteen minutes or more for meditation practice.

Benefits and Systems Being Treated, Challenged, and Healed:

- Stimulates the nervous system and digestive system.

- Meditative and relaxing.

- Increases intuition.

- Spending time with your breathwork will strengthen lungs.

- Opens hips, creating a sense of balance throughout the body.

- Assists in elimination.

- Great pose for meditation.

Precautions and Contraindications:

- Those with pain or tightness in knee, hip joints, or ankles should use modifications.

Yoga Mudra, the Seal of Yoga/Union
SANSKRIT NAME: BADDHA PADMASANA

Does your mind rule your heart? There are times when the mind will not allow what the heart wants to feel. Does your ego overpower the voice of your higher self? Do you know how to let go of the past to forgive yourself and others? When the head bows humbly to the earth, your body and spirit merge, and your intuition awakens, unveiling the wisdom of the divine feminine. As you surrender the will of the mind, the heart opens, coming into alignment and the union of self-love.

Entry and Holding Posture

1. Stand with your feet hip-width apart, the crown of your head lifting up to the sky, shoulder blades squeezing together, chest open and arms at your side.

2. Place your arms behind you with hands interlocked, if possible. Or hold on to a yoga strap, belt, or a man's tie with your hands behind your back.

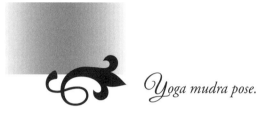

Yoga mudra pose.

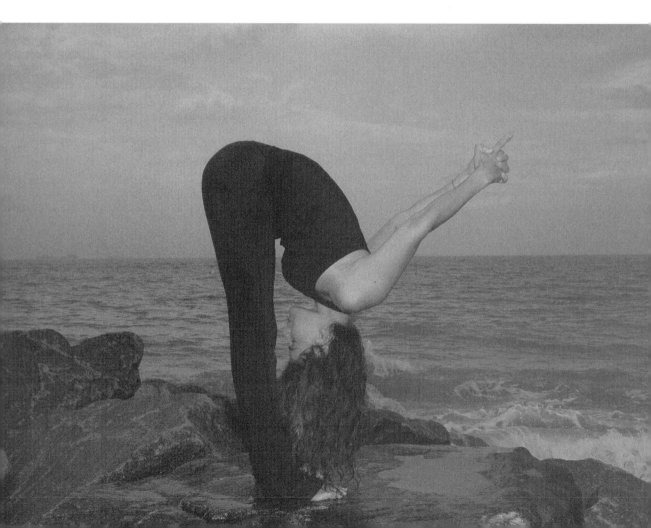

3. Press your hands down toward the ground, lengthening your arms.

4. Slightly bend your knees, pull up on your knee caps, and plant your feet flat on the ground.

5. Slowly, leading with your heart, bring your chest down toward your thighs. Tuck your chin in toward your chest, pull your belly up to your spine, and allow the backs of your legs to lengthen.

6. Breathe in and out through your nostrils only, and feel the opening in your heart.

7. Each exhale of breath, allow yourself to surrender the will and chatter of your mind and come into alignment with your heart.

Hold one to three minutes. If you have high blood pressure, do not hold longer than thirty seconds.

Benefits and Systems Being Treated, Challenged, and Healed:
- Strengthens the immune system.
- Opens the third eye and intuition.
- Balances hormones.
- Aligns the divine will with the physical will.
- Releases serotonin in the brain.
- Compresses internal organs, great for digestion and elimination.
- Compresses kidneys and adrenal glands, releasing stress.
- Strengthens the hamstrings, thighs, shoulders, and triceps.
- Increases blood flow and oxygen to skin and brain for glow and clarity.

Precautions and Contraindications:
- High blood pressure: come out of posture after five breaths or thirty seconds.
- Neck and shoulder injuries: go gently.

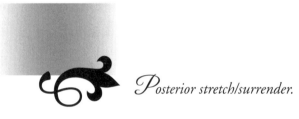 *Posterior stretch/surrender.*

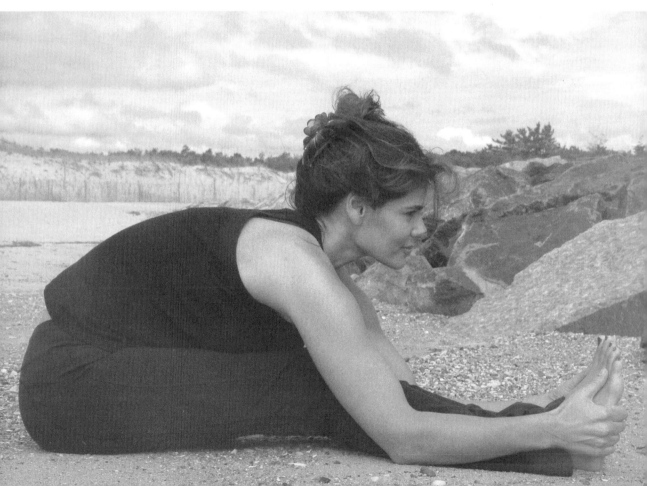

Posterior Stretch/Surrender, or Seated Forward Bend
Sanskrit name: Paschimottanasana

Do you run from your pain? Are you able to feel and look at your pain? Are you holding in or holding back? Can you release and surrender the tension held in the back of your legs and lower back, where the seat of your physical will lies? Relax into this pose and revel in your increased energy and blood flow, which allows you to open to deeper wisdom. This is an exercise of surrendering the heart to forgive yourself and others. In it, your legs are supple yet strong, your mind is open, your head is humbly bowing to the heart, and your heart is surrendering forward. A flexible spine equals a flexible mind. Are you too willful?

Entry and Holding Posture

1. Sit on the ground with your legs straight, your heels pushing forward, and the backs of your knees in contact with the floor.

2. Lift your arms up over your head, palms facing each other, and lengthen through the spine to reach toward the sky.

3. As if your hips were hinged, lengthen your hands toward your feet, bending from your waist with a straight back. Do not allow your belly to cave in.

4. Breathe through your nose with big belly breaths. Allow your breath to do all the work.

5. Tuck your chin into your chest. With each breath, feel your heart surrender, the back of your neck unwind, and your lower back and backs of thighs release tension.

6. Allow yourself to feel what you are holding in or running from. Do not judge; just observe.

7. If you cannot touch your toes, don't worry. Place a pillow under your knees and touch what you can.

Hold one to three minutes. Breathe through the nostrils only.

Benefits and Systems Being Treated, Challenged, and Healed:

- Lengthens and strengthens the spine and hamstrings.

- Opens the lungs for more oxygen and blood flow.

- Relaxes the nervous system by releasing serotonin in the brain.

- Releases pent-up emotions and mental pressure, bringing balance to the mind and relief to the spine.

- Builds fire in the digestive organs and ovaries for digestion and vitality.

- Strengthens and revitalizes the adrenal glands.

- Massages digestive organs.

- Helps elimination.

- Stimulates lymph flow and immune system.

- Sedates nervous system.

- Irrigates kidneys with fresh blood supply.

- Releases toxins.

Precautions and Contraindications:

- Pregnancy, sciatica, and bad backs: use modifications and ease into posture slowly.

Fish/Agility
Sanskrit name: Matsyasana

The fish has the strength and flexibility to move through the water. The fish survives because of its agility. In fish pose, the arch of your spine expands your rib cage like the gills of a fish. Your heart opens, your lungs exhale, releasing a flood of emotions. Your neck bends, the mind relaxes, becoming as flexible as the spine. A flexible spine is a flexible mind. How flexible are you?

Entry and Holding Posture

1. Lie flat, straighten your legs, and flex your toes toward the sky. Placing your hands under your buttocks, palms down, press down on the earth with palms and elbows. Lift your chest and heart toward the sky, and rest the flat part of your head, the top of the crown, on the ground.

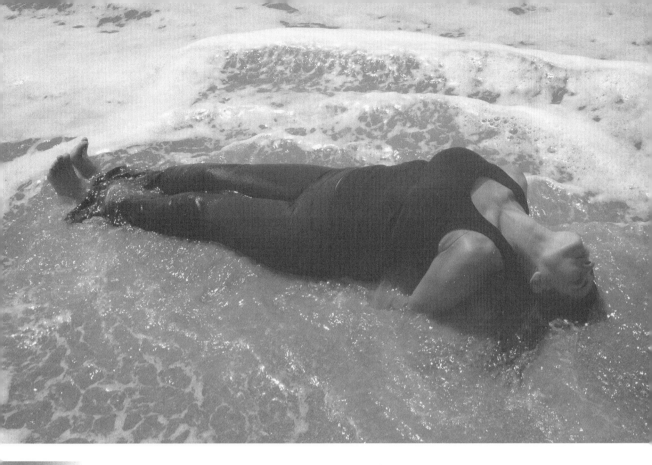

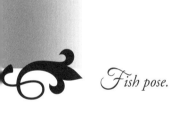 *Fish pose.*

2. Lengthen through your extended legs, engaging the thighs by pressing the backs of your knees into the floor. Your weight and pressure should be evenly distributed on the tailbone and crown of your head.

3. Find your edge of discomfort and hold it there, relaxing and breathing slowly and deeply through your nostrils only into your belly, heart, and throat.

4. Allow the energy to move back and forth from your heart to your throat and third eye.

5. Release by pressing your forearms and palms into the floor; slowly tuck your chin into your chest and roll down one vertebra at a time. Slowly lower yourself down.

6. Draw your knees into your chest and rock slowly from side to side. Focus on integrating wisdom, compassion, and clear communication.

Hold up to 15–30 seconds, or about five big breaths through the nostrils only.

Benefits and Systems Being Treated, Challenged, and Healed:
- Opens the diaphragm and massages the heart muscle and lungs.
- Stimulates the immune system through activation of the thymus.
- Massages and opens the thyroid and parathyroid.
- Opens clear communication.
- Creates compassion in the heart center and clarity in the mind.
- Good for asthma.
- Good for circulatory, respiratory, and immune systems.

Precautions and Contraindications:
- Those with neck or shoulder pain, hyperthyroid, high blood pressure, heart disease or stroke, or low back pain should begin with modifications.

Triangle/Balance
Sanskrit name: Utthita Trikonasana

Do you know where you stand? The triangle is a symbol of strength, unity, balance, and stability. As the arm lengthens and the heart stretches up toward Spirit for spiritual connection, the feet are firmly gripped onto the earth. Can you remain just as grounded in your human self as you evolve in your spiritual self? Can you remain firmly planted in your ideals as your body bends and your heart opens to the divine? Can you feel both forces in balance with each other and working together, your own will and the divine will?

Entry and Holding Posture

Head lifting up toward sky, heart open, squeezing your shoulders, feet hip-width apart and firmly planted into the ground. Hands in prayer at your heart. With an exhalation, step or lightly jump your feet 3½ to 4 feet apart.

1. Raise your arms parallel to the floor and reach them actively out to the sides, shoulder blades wide, palms down.

2. Turn your left foot in slightly to the right and your right foot out to the right 90 degrees. Align the right heel with the left heel. Firm your thighs and turn your right thigh outward, so that the center of the right kneecap is in line with the center of the right ankle.

3. Exhale and extend your torso to the right, directly over the plane of the right leg, bending from the hip joint, not the waist. Anchor this movement by strengthening the left leg and pressing the outer heel firmly to the floor.

4. Rotate the torso to the left, keeping the two sides equally long. Let the left hip come slightly forward and lengthen the tailbone toward the back heel.

5. Rest your right hand on your shin, ankle, or the floor outside your right foot, whatever is possible without distorting the sides of the torso.

6. Stretch your left arm toward the ceiling, in line with the tops of your shoulders. Keep your head in a neutral position or turn it to the left, eyes gazing softly at the left thumb.

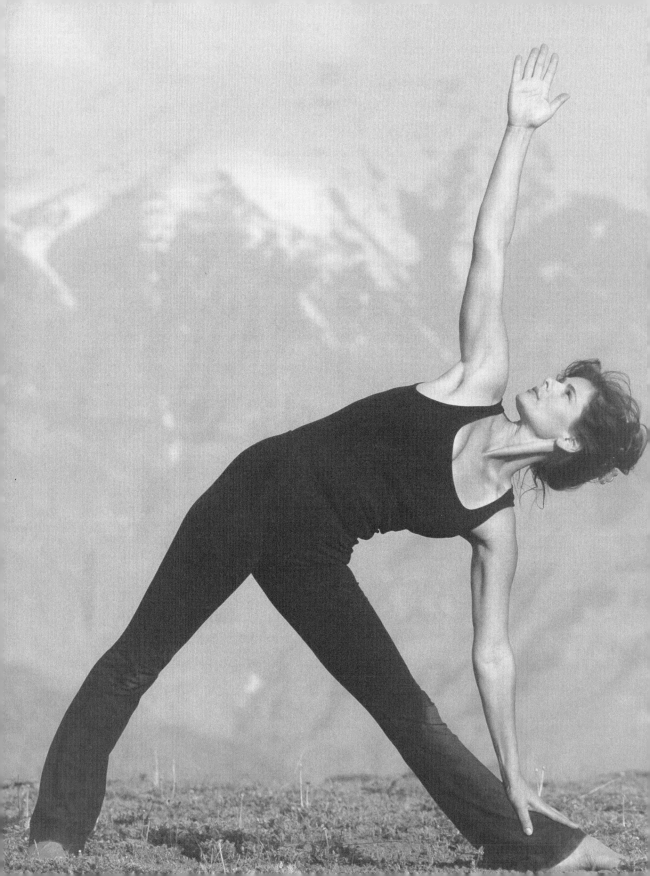

7. Inhale to come up, strongly pressing the back heel into the floor and reaching the top arm toward the ceiling.

8. Reverse the feet and repeat for the same length of time to the left.

Hold up to 15–30 seconds each side, or about five big breaths through the nostrils only.

Benefits and Systems Being Treated, Challenged, and Healed:

- Opens chest and spine.

- Stimulates abdominal glands.

- Relieves stress.

- Improves digestion.

- Helps relieve symptoms of menopause.

- Relieves backache.

- Therapeutic for flat feet, neck pain, osteoporosis, and sciatica.

- Stimulates the abdominal organs.

- Opens hips, groin, hamstrings, and calves.

- Strengthens thighs, knees, and ankles.

Precautions and Contraindications:

- Low blood pressure

- Diarrhea

- Headache

- Heart condition: Practice against a wall. Keep the top arm on the hip.

- High blood pressure: Turn your head to gaze downward in the final pose.

- Neck problems: Don't turn your head to look upward; continue looking straight ahead and keep both sides of the neck evenly long.

Triangle pose.

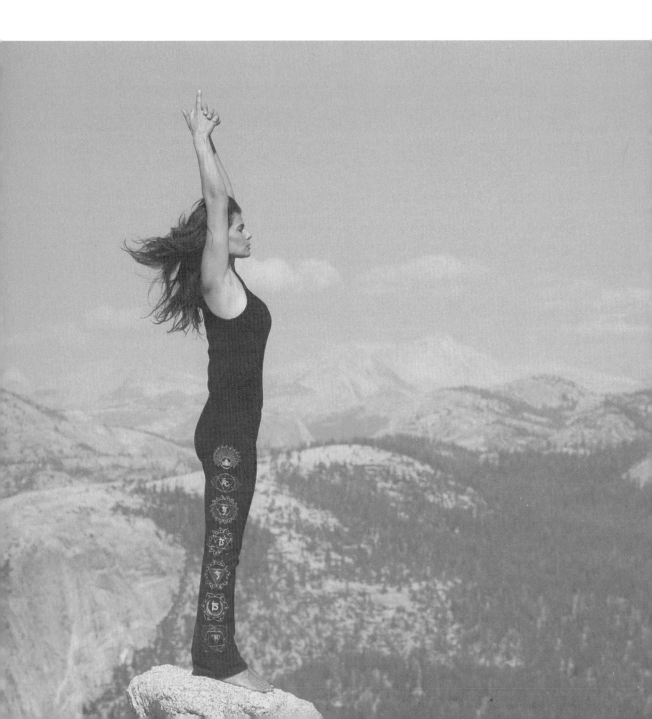

Chapter 3

THE MENTAL BODY

Health and happiness are often the result of choices we consciously make with our mind. But many times, an overactive mind does not allow for what the heart truly wants to feel. Every day, as you go about your work and your life, you are fundamentally choosing between fear or faith—fear of the unknown and faith that you are on track and doing things right. Both fear and faith are unseen forces. Which one do you choose? Where will your energy go?

Years ago, in my heart I knew I had to follow my true path, but my mind would not allow my emotions to flow freely for fear of them being too much to handle—until my near-death experience (or what I now jokingly refer to as my two-by-four-to-the-head wake-up call), when all my emotions rose up to the top. That situation taught me how my true power comes from trusting my heart and taking the time to stop, look, and listen so that I could feel my life instead of trying to control it.

Belief systems come from our environment—our culture, family, religion, society, world, economy, education systems, media, and everything that surrounds us. They are the seeds that are planted in our minds and hearts that either take us closer to our higher, true self or further away from it. Belief systems form the thought patterns that

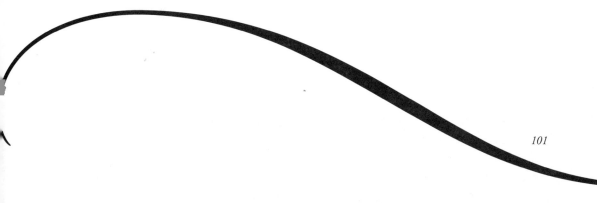

can grow strong and beautiful like a flower that radiates color, life, perfume, and balance—or can become a weed that feeds off the life force and radiance of others because it does not know how to hold its own space and radiate its own life force.

My experience as a young girl growing up in a religious family disrupted and confused my innate system of beliefs. When I was a little girl, I remember how connected I felt to God. I did not have a name for Spirit, but I knew in my bones that it existed. I felt that God was everywhere and in everything—trees, animals, people, and even the school desk and chair I sat on. I was very content with my understanding and connection to God—until my first day of confession (or, as I call it, my first day of confusion).

I was in CCD (Catholic Sunday school), and I hated it. I fought my parents tooth and nail every Sunday—my day to run free and connect with *my* God through nature. But instead, I was forced to sit down and listen to stories *about* God. It was not that I did not like the other children or didn't want to learn something new; I just did not want to learn what they were teaching. It made me rebellious, and in turn, I was punished by the nuns with the dreaded ruler.

I remember feeling lost and confused: Why did my parents force me to go? How could they believe in this stuff? It was such a contradiction to what I knew from my own experience. Yet I was forced to continue my CCD school so I could be confirmed—a Catholic ritual that demonstrates you are part of the community now. But I did not want to be part of this God.

In the process of the ritual, I had to go to confession. I remember being first in line and walking down the aisle of the church. A priest told me to stop at this old-looking phone booth that looked like it had prison bars on it. He then directed me to step in and close the curtain behind me. I then heard a deep man's voice coming through the bars, asking me to tell my sins. I did not know at the time what that really meant—I was only eight years old, after all. He prompted me to tell him about any bad things I had done, such as hit my siblings, say a bad word, or talk back to my parents. I thought to myself, "I know a lot of adults who should be sitting here, but I do not know of any bad things I have done." I was not a willing participant in this game of tattletale. The priest was losing patience with me.

He then proceeded to tell me that if I did not confess my sins to him, I would be a sinner, and he and God would not like me because I behaved badly. I thought to myself for a brief moment, and in that one moment of silence, my native wisdom came forth. Here is what it said, and what I relayed to the priest:

"I do not understand. My God is everywhere and everything. Why do I need you to talk to God? I do this talking to the trees and the animals, and in my prayers at night before I go to bed. I do not fear my God. And why is he always considered a man? Why is it that I am supposed to fear God and Santa Claus, when they are supposed to love me?" Let's just say this innate wisdom had a tongue that definitely got me into trouble and my parents an earful.

When I left the confessional, I felt fear and doubt in my mind and heart about God. I felt punished for my own wisdom. The belief system I was being forced to swallow killed the most precious muscles of my mind—my clarity, trust, and ability to see and talk to my God. This is where the first seed was planted in my mind and heart that took me further away from God and my higher self.

Here's another, more beautiful story that involves my father and how he instilled a strong value system in me. He was an exceptional athlete. He played semi-professional baseball, golf, and tennis. He loved sports so much, he coached Little League in his spare time. Since I was his first child, the oldest of four, he took me to all his practices. My father never said I couldn't play on a team or get dirty because I was a girl. At the age of five, I was a bat girl for his boys' baseball team. And by the age of eight, I was the first girl on the boys' baseball team. There were very few team sports for girls back in the 1970s.

My dad recognized my athletic abilities and encouraged me all the way. By the time I was fifteen, I was playing fast-pitch softball for a New Jersey semi-pro team. I then went to college on a softball scholarship. My dad was so proud of my talents. He never said I couldn't do something because I was a girl. If anything, he loved to see me beat the boys. He would tell the boys on his team, "Have no mercy on her, because she will have no mercy on you." He taught me focus, discipline, commitment, and perseverance. His encouragement helped make me who I am today and prepared me to do what I do. He saw my talents and fully supported who I was. He helped create the Goddess Warrior within me by giving me the strong belief that it was good to be a righteous, truthful woman who knew her strengths and had no fear of her power.

My distrust of God—the seed of which was planted in that confessional—stayed with me until my dance with death. My wake-up call was losing a child, but yours could come from many instances, such as cancer or other illness, a death in the family, a car accident, or any trauma that shakes you and awakens you. My near-death experience shifted my perception and put me back into alignment with my higher self and my inborn intelligence that I am a creature of God and one with all of creation. This experience put me back in alignment with what I already knew at eight years old. It validated everything I knew as a child, and I knew that I would never doubt my God or myself again.

Our experiences teach us to either listen to our inner voice or to stuff it down. Here is another story from my past that illustrates how the mental body operates. I share it in the hope that you might be able to see yourself in this story and realize how your mental body might be contributing to your own unhappiness.

When I was a young girl, I was sexually abused. I put all memory of and feelings about the experience in a box, hoping they would never show their ugly head. I never spoke of it until I went to therapy. And after my near-death experience, everything I had ever stuffed down came flowing back up again. It was only then that I realized I had never really gotten rid of the pain—instead, I had been unknowingly reminding myself of it by punishing myself with many bad habits, negative thoughts, personality conflicts, and masks that I wore to protect myself from a world I did not trust.

Growing up, I had a good reason not to trust or love men; I had a love-hate relationship with them. This experience of sexual abuse was a betrayal to my spirit. But it would also become the savior of my soul, because it gave me the opportunity to choose not to be a victim any longer. I chose to seek the truth, and when I did, as ugly as it was, it released me from the prison cell that I had gotten so accustomed to.

When I dug deep into the depths of my own soul, I healed not only myself but also the dysfunction that had been passed down from one generation to the next in my family tree. We are each destined to repeat the actions of our parents and ancestors—good and bad, fortunate and unfortunate—until someone in our family is strong enough to stand up to the old patterns, belief systems, and dysfunctions. It is the law of energy, the law of life. You may come from an alcoholic background and may never have picked up a drink or you may have your own problem with alcohol. Regardless of your consumption, you have the same behaviors and beliefs that your family does: you likely do not follow through or complete tasks, you do not trust others, you fear intimacy. Whether or not you have an alcoholic lifestyle, you have an alcoholic belief system that has become ingrained in you. This law of energy is true for any dysfunction.

When you choose to truly heal yourself, you must ask yourself how much you want to heal. How deep do you want to go? How much do you want to know and look at?

How much do you truly love yourself? And are you powerful enough to plumb the core of your existence for yourself and for your children? You must always remember that people treat you the way you *allow* them to treat you. You choose whether you are a victim of life or a participant in it, because if you cannot love yourself, how can you teach self-love to your children and to others? When I chose to go deep with my healing, my pain was also deep. And so was the relief when I realized that what I knew, saw, and experienced was real and not my imagination, and that my instincts and intuition were always correct. I also validated my own female ancestors, who I later found out had also been abused. I learned that their stories were similar to mine. This is why I ask every woman who attends Boot Camp for Goddesses the following questions: Who are the past three generations of women on your mother's side? Do you know their maiden names? Where they went to school? *If* they went to school? What they did with their lives? Their story is your story.

The natives say when you heal yourself, you also heal the four generations before and the four generations after you. I can tell you this is true. I have five nieces who now have a brighter future since these old behaviors have come to light. And my sister, mother, grandmothers, and female cousins have all healed from the core of this truth. We all support each other and love each other, and there is no blame and no drama. We have learned to respect the goddess in each of us and have set this example for my nieces.

You have to decide to stop turning your pain and anger against yourself, and give yourself permission to love yourself. As I often remind myself, "I would rather be led by my heart than ruled by my mind." True love has energy, force, and action behind it. It weaves together the spiritual and mental bodies. There is nothing more validating and freeing than to deem yourself worthy of your own love. When you no longer look for love outside of yourself, you will know that you *are* love, and you will attract love abundantly from near and far.

This is the power of belief systems—thoughts, attitudes, and, most of all, choices can save your and others' lives or be the death of both your and the next generation's spirit and soul. You must remember that experiences—no matter how painful—are only things that have *happened* to you. They are not who you are at the core unless you allow them to be. This fundamental truth is the message of Sophia, the goddess of wisdom, that helped and ultimately saved me. The old saying that the truth shall set you free is true in every sense.

Goddess of the Mental Body:
SOPHIA, GODDESS OF WISDOM

Sophia is present in numerous cultures: she is called Sophia in Greek, Hokhma in Hebrew, Sapientia in Latin, Sheela-na-gig in Celtic. There were temples built to her all over the ancient world. Her shrine in Istanbul, Hagia Sophia, is regarded as the eighth wonder of the world.

Sophia is considered to be the mother of God in the Judeo-Christian tradition. Almost everyone is familiar with the painting by Michelangelo on the ceiling of the Sistine Chapel. It is a depiction of God reaching out with his finger to touch Adam's finger. At least that is the image that always comes to mind. In that iconic painting, Sophia is on God's other side. Although Sophia is in plain sight, we only notice God and Adam. Isn't that interesting?

A Sophia woman has no fear of the truth. She sees it all and tells it as it is. She brings meaning to human experience with her gift of understanding "the bigger picture."

Descriptors
FOR THIS GODDESS

Wise, loving, communicative, knowledgeable, creative, protective, giving, truthful

Message from This Goddess[16]

From the moment you enter the world until the time you surrender to death, all that you experience directly for yourself—all the burnt fingers to discover that fire is hot, all the falling flat when your reach exceeds your grasp, all the explorations of territory known and unknown—are pathways to me. Seek to know, and you are me. Stretch to become, and you are me. The feminine quests for wisdom. The feminine is part of all women. All women have wisdom. All women are me.

I give you my three daughters, Faith, Hope, and Charity, as gifts that can help you overcome the despair, confusion, and suffering that frame human life. I urge you to remember that clear vision and understanding line the path that leads to the discovery of the meaning of your life. Only when you stand back, gaining some emotional distance, can you see that even the most traumatic experiences can be the birthplace

---

16   Used with permission from Amy Sophia Marashinsky's *The Goddess Oracle* (U.S. Games Systems, 2006).

of your most treasured strengths. It is only in times of great stress that heroic feats are truly appreciated.

How This Goddess Works in Your Life

Each one of us has a story to tell, a story of how our innate wisdom has helped us or saved us. We also all have stories of times when we have shut down or shut up this inner wisdom because of fear of the truth.

Women have been silenced for fear of our power, yet today we have to learn the strength of being silent so we are able to hear our intuition, our most powerful gift and tool. Remember that as a culture, we are told to go to our rooms and sit in a corner in silence, so how could you think being silenced is not a punishment?

How many times have you shut up to make someone else more comfortable? Many of us realize too late the consequences of not listening to our inner wisdom. We are conditioned to be silent—not in a powerful way of listening to our intuition and spirit, but to be silenced for fear of the truth. Listen to a little girl for a day and hear how her wisdom shines through her voice, filled with inspiration and enthusiasm. She sees and hears things that others cannot. She wonders if she is crazy for these thoughts and clarity because no one else can sense them.

The problem is she *is* right on, she *is* tuned in, but others around her most often are tuned out. Sophia is within her and still to this day is in every woman. We have just stopped listening to her words of wisdom for fear of confrontation, change, or being different, which means the ultimate fear: standing alone. The most powerful words of wisdom I have heard from my inner Sophia and still follow to this day are these: *When you stand in your power, which is your wisdom, your suffering will stop.* This has been my mantra for decades, and I am never alone. I have more love and abundance of health, wealth, and success because I follow my inner voice and truth.

How many times have you looked at the potential of things instead of the reality of the situation? How many times have you silenced your inner voice to allow the fantasy of the situation to rise instead of the truth of the matter? For instance, you might have had the experience of falling in love with the potential of a man instead of the reality of who he is. When you met him, you knew Sophia was talking to you, but you silenced her because you did not want to see the truth. Years later, you have two kids, a marriage that ended in a divorce, and are fighting for what is legally yours, all because you did not listen. You settled our of fear of being alone or not feeling able to protect or financially support yourself.

This sort of thing also happens in our families. Sometimes, an entire family can be stuck in a pattern of dysfunction while you are working to free yourself. Your family members try to pull back into the tribal energy of the dysfunction, and you feel like a salmon swimming upstream and out of unhealthy waters. You have awakened, and it is your responsibility to follow through if you want to be free. This may be a lonely place, but were you not alone, feeling isolated or different in the first place? May this truth and realization ignite the fire of anger and pain yet put you back into alignment with your inner Sophia and voice of God. Remember, Faith and Hope are Sophia's daughters, your best friends and the inner wisdom of God/Goddess.

What Is the Mental Body?

The mental body is ruled by the air element. The wind is the breath of Mother Earth. Like the spiritual body, the mental body is intangible and nondimensional. It is a place of magic and mystery, where the mind conducts thought, stores knowledge, and builds intellect and wisdom based on internal and external stimuli.

The mental body is where our innate wisdom lies—wisdom we were born with and wisdom we have learned from experiences during our journey of life. This inner wisdom is the driving force that is constantly challenging us to move closer to our higher self, work toward our true potential, and connect with Spirit. This native wisdom possesses the infinite knowledge of how the universe works—the mystery and magic of how all things are connected. We each have a craving to connect to this knowledge, to try and make sense of it all, yet we already know how the universe works. It is embedded in our cells and imprinted in our hearts. As a human being, our purpose is to use all of our senses to taste, see, smell, hear, and feel this reality in order to reawaken the wisdom that already resides within.

We learn how to tap in and access this wisdom through experience. As we acquire knowledge, we build the ability to understand and profit from experience. With every experience, our intelligence makes choices that either take us closer to Truth or further away. It all depends on our thoughts, belief systems, values, attitude, focus, intentions, masks, ego, personality, inner wisdom, intelligence, and choice. The power to choose is a

God-given gift of the mind, yet it can also be one of the most detrimental tools we have. The mind is a powerful tool or your worst enemy; it all depends on how you use it.

Muscles of the Mental Body

Thought

The power of thought is the power of creation. A thought is whatever arises in the mind, a symbolic response to stimuli. A thought may be an idea, an image, a sound, a smell, a touch, or even an emotional feeling that arises from the brain. It is an unexplainable force—energy that can either be your savior or your worst enemy, depending on how you perceive, filter, download, and access the information.

A thought is a wave of information that comes into the mind like a cloud passing in the sky. Studies have shown that the average person has 50,000 thoughts a day. But thoughts don't exist independently from the others; they cluster in patterns so that we don't have to discern each thought from each other. It's these thought patterns that create judgment, which separates good from evil and results in belief systems.

How you think determines how you feel; how you feel determines how you behave; and how you behave determines what you create.

Belief System

A belief system is a thought pattern that has been created in our minds as a result of stimuli and experiences. It is a set of rules we abide by consciously and unconsciously to help decide what we want to do with the information our minds are constantly gathering. A belief system is a means of gathering, manipulating, storing, retrieving, and classifying recorded information. In a moment of reflection, the mind compares a new experience to a stored experience and makes a judgment about the new experience. This act of judgment creates a belief system. A belief system will either create fear and doubt or it will reinforce trust and truth.

Belief systems are not only stored in the mind—over time, they take up residence in our nervous system, organs, glands, muscles, and tissues. Your fight-or-flight response is dependent on your belief systems. They help you decide, do I stay and fight for this cause or do I flee because it is not worth my time or energy? Is this good or evil, safe or unsafe? The brain processes this information, trying to recognize it as something pleasurable or painful. Once the brain makes its judgment, it will tell the body to either move deeper into this experience or further away. The mind will always move away from discomfort in order to keep you safe. We all prefer to do things we like—what we are good at and what makes us feel good. In yoga, I used to hate doing all the hip openers because all it did was bring up pain. I hated seeing a baby because it brought up my pain. I could not smell a certain cologne because it brought flashbacks of my abuse.

It can be extremely challenging to heal belief systems until we are able to truly see where they came from. Only when we can look at them without judgment—which creates separation, guilt, and shame—can we determine if the belief system is helping us or hurting us. Does it take you to the core of your being and true nature or does it distract you and, in the long run, hurt you?

When we can bring balance to the intuitive and intellectual parts of our brain, we can erase the belief systems we no longer want or need, as if erasing a chalkboard. It creates more space in your mind, which then creates more space and flexibility in your body. When we function from a new awareness and insight, intelligence goes beyond the intellectual.

Intelligence

Intelligence is the ability to understand and profit from experience by acquiring, storing, sorting, and applying knowledge. There are many types of intelligence: emotional intelligence, mathematical intelligence, creative intelligence, scientific intelligence, and healing intelligence, to name a few. Yet there are two fundamental forms of intelligence: book intelligence and innate, natural body intelligence, also known as holistic intelligence.

Our culture only seems to reward book intelligence. Book intelligence brings power, prestige, and money. If you do not have this intelligence, you will most likely be unsuccessful, no matter what you do. You will suffer without book intelligence, so go out there and get a degree.

Our approach to intelligence is very linear; we often choose to believe only what we can prove to be true. We are, for the most part, closed off to one of the most crucial types of intelligence that every human being has: the innate intelligence that resides in every cell of our being, which knows we are all natives to Mother Earth. "Native" means we are children of our creator, God, the Great Spirit, who lives upon and with Mother Earth. We typically think "native" refers to particular cultures, such as Native Americans, Australian Aborigines, or indigenous tribes such as the Shipibo of the Amazon, but "native" actually means a person who belongs to a particular place. And we, each and every one of us, possess the knowledge that we belong and are connected to Mother Earth.

Where did our culture and others lose this native intelligence, and why? As we talked about, most religions, countries, and societies have diminished the feminine essence of God, which is manifest in Mother Nature. Our need for book intelligence has outweighed our innate need for harmony and balance. In order to be whole, holy, and healthy, we must give equal power to both aspects of life, energy and ourselves—the masculine and the feminine—in order to be truly powerful.

The ancient native tribes never lost their connection to the feminine, yet we punished, even killed, many of them because we looked at them as savages. We denigrated their relationship to Mother Nature and Spirit, their instincts, and their intuition. To relearn this inborn intelligence, we all have to go to the bare essentials in order to move forward. Instead of depleting Mother Earth of her resources and slaughtering those who live in harmony with her, we need to face and end our own self-violence, no matter how big or small. When we are ready to go deeper and find this intelligence within, believe me, Spirit will come knocking. And when it does happen, if you are willing to do the work, it will release you, heal you, and bring you back into alignment with your body and heart as a whole and holy person. If are willing to do the work, you will find the missing pieces of your fragmented self, like putting a puzzle together. Every piece of information is a gift, a clue that guides you to find the ultimate treasure—your authentic, native, natural, and pure self.

All the pain and suffering in the world now is only a reflection of what we have chosen as a race, and now we need to take responsibility for those past choices. We must be willing to walk through the fire and face our fears head-on to relieve this pain. Our spirits are hearing the call as if the bugle were blowing to go to war. But this war is an internal war, calling forth the spiritual warrior in order to find peace and self-love. You can either surrender to the calling or choose to get hit over the head (metaphorically) with a two-by-four. The choice is always yours; how deep do you want to go?

When you face your inner demons, you develop a spiritual muscle that enables you to become one with your enemy—which, in most cases, is yourself. This spiritual muscle puts the mental body to work, just as if you were doing reps in the gym with weights. I call this doing mental push-ups—training the mental body to face the pain and move through it instead of running away from it. This is the purpose of ritual and ceremony—to put us back into harmony with Spirit and Mother Earth. This is the intelligence of the native people around the world, and also of everyone and everything God has created. Are you ready for the shaman's death? Or, to rephrase, are you ready to surrender your fears and step up to the plate, work to your true potential, and live from your authentic self? Are you ready to stop complaining about life and start creating change? These are the questions of the native intelligence. The answers will be found once you take the first step, to surrender what is no longer of service to you. This is the wisdom that women yearn for and have forgotten and all human beings are craving.

My own personal daily prayer is to kneel in honor of Mother Earth and say one of two things: "May I know my truth, may I see my truth, may I speak my truth, may I feel my truth; O Great Spirit, give me the strength, perseverance, and courage to follow you and my path. *Aho*." Or, "May my eyes, ears, and heart be open to receive you, O Great Spirit. Please get this lesson over with as soon as possible, and please have mercy and compassion on me. *Aho*." In other words, please show me the way, but be gentle.

This native intelligence is beyond our consciousness. It is the mystery and magic of the universe. One familiar saying that we all hear is "We are all one." It's so simple, yet so complex. As women, we are one step closer to this native intelligence because we carry the same gifts—strength, compassion, and native intelligence—as Mother Earth. It is in every ounce of our being. That is why we are the true healers.

Our culture as a whole is suffering from many diseases, such as depression, obesity, eating disorders, ADD, and addictions, all because our education and religious systems deny us the ability to tap into our own inborn intelligence. We pressure our children to learn more and more, to the point where most of their time is spent with their head in a book or in front of a computer screen. The pressure of this emphasis has steep consequences, such as suicide, peer pressure, addiction, and an overconsumption of sex. We are raising our children to be successful instead of becoming functional and fulfilled human beings. When we foster our holistic intelligence, we are in harmony with the universal flow and will naturally attract an abundance of love, health, wealth, and success.

It is no wonder that all the patriarchal systems—political, religious, and educational—are failing: they never gave equal weight to book intelligence and inborn intelligence. They are based on creating fear instead of love. If you do not confess your sins, you will be doomed; if you are a woman, you have fewer rights and less value than a man—you have to work all your life just to get by; women do not deserve to be educated because their only true purpose is to have babies. There are so many rules and regulations that bring fear into our lives instead of the most powerful intelligence of all: love.

Education and religion teach us to work from the outside in—to prove our intelligence with tests and to build temples and churches so that we can connect to God. Natural intelligence works from the inside out. We are each born with an inner knowing of how the universe works. It gives us the ability to heal on all levels—spiritual, mental, emotional, and physical.

Left and Right Brain

The two different types of intelligence stem from the two different sides of our brain. When the gifts of both sides of our intelligence come together, when we can balance the holistic body intelligence with the external educational intelligence, we can create power, peace, wholeness, and holiness.

The left brain controls the muscles on the right side of the body. It rules the masculine aspects of self, including intellect, force, math, logic, analytic ability, and ego. The left brain is also the seat of language, and it works in a very ordered, linear fashion.

The right brain controls the left side of the body and governs the feminine aspects of self—the intuitive, allowing, creative, and fluid self. The right side is more visual and processes intuitively, holistically, and randomly.

Over time, the left brain has become dominant. We have trained our brains to be in a constant state of doing and producing, but not being. This stresses us mentally by constantly putting our brain and our body on overload and triggering the fight-or-flight response. This imbalance closes off our ability to breathe fully into our lungs, and it shuts down the most important natural medicine produced by our bodies—serotonin. Serotonin creates peace and stillness in our hearts and minds; it soothes the nervous system and helps us open up to our intuition. Over time, a lack of serotonin in the brain can lead to depression, ADD, and addictions, whether they be related to food, weight, drugs, alcohol, or sex.

Only when we can look at both sides of an issue can we reach a balanced decision. If we continue to only think with the left side of our brains, we will constantly be reacting to situations, creating more havoc and chaos and more karma that keeps us lost in a maze. We never get the point of our existence unless we can go full circle in all aspects of our being: spiritually, mentally, emotionally, and physically.

Serotonin

Serotonin is a neurotransmitter involved in the transmission of nerve impulses. It promotes feelings of happiness and is believed to regulate our moods, help with sleep, calm anxiety, and relieve depression.

Your body makes serotonin out of the amino acid tryptophan. Low levels of serotonin are associated with depression, anxiety, apathy, fear, feelings of worthlessness, insomnia, and fatigue. We are learning that depression is related to a number of other health issues—the National Institute of Mental Health considers depression a risk factor for high blood pressure, high cholesterol, and heart disease. Depression is the nation's most prevalent mental health problem, affecting about 15 million Americans, who spend about $3 billion a year on drugs to battle it.[17] Almost all of these medicines target either serotonin or norepinephrine, another important neurotransmitter.

Our diet, thoughts, emotions, behavior, and connection to nature all affect our body chemistry. Relaxation, exercise, breathing, and good nutrition all have a positive impact on our bodies' chemical processes. It is possible to use these techniques to manage your body's serotonin levels. When you pay attention to the little things that make you feel good and systematically include them in your daily routine, you encourage your body to manage its levels of serotonin. Just getting out of bed and into a warm shower elevates serotonin levels, making it easier to get into a positive, constructive frame of mind. We know, instinctively, that pampering ourselves creates a feeling of well-being, but we often keep ourselves so busy that we "don't have the time" to sit still in pleasant surroundings, listen to our favorite music, eat nutritious food, or spend quality time with loved ones on a daily basis.

Ego

Just as God has many manifestations—including goddesses, angels, animals, nature, and spirit guides—so does the ego self, with masks, split personalities, and inner demons, or as I call them, the itty-bitty shitty committee. The ego is your inner critic. It is the internal voice that will churn out stories and beliefs to keep the heart from feeling what it wants to feel. The ego often plays a large role in which belief systems hold sway over

---

17   See http://www.angelfire.com/hi/TheSeer/seratonin.html.

your mind. A belief system will either feed the ego self by reinforcing fear and doubt or it will feed the higher self, which will build a strong foundation and sense of self.

The ego is the part of ourselves that has lost its way. It is the voice of terror that puts your body in constant a state of fight-or-flight. It is a part of our lower self that is selfish, willful, defensive, impatient, and closed off to feeling. The ego self tells you that you are not good enough, that you don't deserve good things, and it keeps you from envisioning a brighter and more fulfilling future. The ego fears death and separates itself from Spirit to create its own identity, leading to judgment and competition. When you find yourself comparing yourself to others, favorably or unfavorably, it is the ego mind at work.

The ego thinks it is the supreme power, in control of your mind and your body, and it idolizes itself. It is afraid to give up, whether it be surrendering an old belief system or surrendering to death itself. The ego mind manipulates the mind as a whole to create judgment. It creates belief systems that will support its own survival. It can reprogram the mind and wipe out your inner wisdom if you allow it to, just like a virus can infect your computer. Once a belief system is embedded in your cellular makeup, it can take over the vibration of your bodies and alter your very existence. You can lose touch with your divine spark. The ego will hail itself and turn your mind into a vehicle of self-destruction, creating disease, addiction, codependency, and more—all to keep you from becoming your divine, authentic self.

The ego loves to waste your time and energy by keeping you in a state of chaos and confusion. Why? The ego needs to be heard, validated, and in control. It will beat you and betray you every time unless you learn how to validate it in a healthy, conscious way and give it a constructive job instead of a destructive one.

The Ego: Friend or Foe?

The ego is like a maze in that it never wants you to see where you are going. By contrast, your higher self is like a labyrinth—you can always see the center, and you will definitely get there if you are willing to follow the path. The maze keeps you confused and irritable, while the labyrinth cultivates trust and peace. (You can see how all things are connected—the labyrinth, DNA, kundalini energy, and the snake are all represented by the spiral, a never-ending, self-energizing force that radiates from the inside out.)

A mouse in a maze is constantly, chaotically looking for a way out. Fear outweighs reason, the senses are overstimulated, the nervous system is overloaded, and the mouse runs into walls and injures itself in a frantic search to get out. Perhaps the mouse will find its way out, but will it be worth the pain and trauma? The ego works the same way. It puts you in a constant state of fight-or-flight and hurls injurious thoughts and beliefs at you to keep you bewildered. If you have 50,000 thoughts a day and you hear "I'm not worthy" enough times, it is no wonder the higher self is drowned out. The ego will risk your physical, mental, emotional, and spiritual health before it will let you think you can get rid of it.

The ego will desensitize your heart and fog your mind, taking you out of your body and into the abyss of fear, where you fall prey to the paralysis of analysis that I call mind masturbation. It will numb out your instincts and intuition in order to be in control. The ego is a type-A personality that will run you into the ground unless you learn how to shut it up and put it in its place.

For women, the ego constantly tells us to sacrifice our own well-being in order to help others—a belief system that has been around for thousands of years. If you think you are free from or unaffected by this subtle voice, think again. Ask yourself why addiction is so prevalent in our culture; why one out of four women are sexually abused; why our children and the average American are overweight; why depression is so common. Will your ego even allow you to truly feel the significance and the ramifications of these statistics?

When the ego gets so strong it separates your higher self into scattered pieces, you become fragmented. In this state, you no longer know your core or feel grounded and connected to anyone, including Spirit and Mother Earth. You become isolated. This fragmentation creates new belief systems, and they become so strong they create their own traits, which then solidify into personalities, or masks, that distort and hide your inner divine spark.

There is hope that you can defeat your own worst enemy—your ego—by learning and practicing the exercises for a healthy mental body.

Personality and Split Personalities

Personality is defined as a dynamic and organized set of characteristics possessed by a person that uniquely influences his or her thoughts, motivations, and behaviors in various situations. The word *personality* originates from the Latin *persona*, which means "mask." The personality can take on more than one face, or mask, and become split personalities. A belief system can also take on its own personality and mask, becoming a concrete part of the human psyche and working to create our reality.

The purpose of the personality is to mirror the divine light that shines through our eyes and radiates through our body like a light. When we lose that shine, the personality will take on many masks to protect itself from the outside world.

Mask

A mask is an artifact normally worn on the face, typically for protection, concealment, performance, or amusement. This is the first definition that most people think of when they hear the word. Yet in the world of the mind it can refer to something entirely different—a persona that is a construct of the ego mind.

A mask is an unauthentic self, a fake. It is negative, defensive, out of touch with the higher self, isolated from others, and under enormous amounts of pressure to keep up the façade.

The mask-self voices such internal comments as

> *I'll reject you before you reject me*
> *I don't need you; I don't need anyone*
> *Yes, but...*

When a personality no longer can identify itself as being an expression of the divine, it is led by the ego to create a mask to protect the individual from the outside world. The mask then becomes a physical expression of unexpressed emotions and thoughts.

THE FIRST TIME I SAW MY MASK

When I was younger, the belief system I created in my mind was that men were not to be trusted; they all wanted to hurt me. Pretty powerful stuff, but it has to be strong and fearful for the ego self to believe it. I created this belief system from the stimuli I received from my experience of being sexually abused in order to protect myself.

Every time I saw a man—even my father, grandfathers, uncles, and cousins—my first reaction was fear that they would hurt me. Every time I saw a man, I had bad thoughts and feelings about him and about myself, because I also felt shame and guilt. As I grew older, I felt angry and sad that I couldn't trust men. I wanted to be close to them but could not trust them, because my belief system said they would betray me. The feelings of wanting to be close to other humans was the inborn intelligence of my mind and body. Yet every time I felt excited or good about a boy or man in my life, I quickly replaced those good feelings with anger and sadness, because how could I allow myself to become close to a male when all men were potentially harmful?

The anger built as I got older, as did the belief system. I wanted to control men instead of them controlling me. I thought I was in control by controlling them through my sexuality. But the truth is that I was totally out of control and giving away my power. The feelings of helplessness and confusion were masked by my anger and my wanting to hurt them before they hurt me.

I remember getting all dressed up to go out one evening and putting on my makeup as if it were war paint. I realized I was painting my face as if it were a mask. I was amazed to see how much I could transform myself with makeup and clothing. Did I want to be a vixen or a shy little girl? It was all about numbing out my higher self in order to find a partner at any cost. I was swallowing my emotions and hiding my true beauty for fear of feeling weak. I continually hurt myself with toxic thoughts so my belief system would be right: *I wasn't good enough; I didn't deserve good things; men were only something to fear, not something to love.* These beliefs grew like cancer. (And we wonder what causes disease.) It got so bad that I had eating disorders, addiction problems, and failed relationships.

The ego self always threw up red flags when I felt emotion, like the robot in *Lost in Space* that shouts, "Danger! Danger!" This loss of emotion gave my ego and belief systems even more power. Although my higher self longed to connect with a partner, my ego only wanted to conquer the enemy—men. In my heart, I never hated men, but my ego feared love and intimacy. My mind would not allow what my heart wanted to feel. If you look at how the mind works, it has many powerful assets that can heal us or destroy us. The great part is what we create, we can also disassemble.

My personality took on a life of its own and learned how to wear many masks, or split personalities. Each personality had its own belief systems, such as: *be nice; you are only to be seen, not heard; your worth is derived only by your looks.* In my mind, I never felt good or worthy, so I created a belief system that said if I can look pretty, maybe I can hide my valuelessness.

Split personalities can become visible through the mask we wear. They are just belief systems you have taken on to help you relate to others and the outside world. They take on many traits to help you manipulate any situation to get what you need at any given moment.

When I finally realized that I was creating my reality through this one belief system, I had to look at where the seed was planted and start pulling some weeds. I knew that if I didn't go through the painful process of really seeing what I was thinking, my future would be grim—addiction, alcoholism, abusive relationships, and prostitution can all arise from the belief that all men are bad. I needed to create a new story with new players. I learned that when you face your pain, there is fear—but there is also relief. A part of you is dying slowly every day; why not walk through the fire and face it? I chose to listen to the newer, truer version of myself that was waiting to be rebirthed.

What we have done as women is become chameleons instead of goddesses. We have taken on masks that have distorted ourselves and our feminine essence. Next time you get dressed and look yourself in the mirror, see if you can identify your mask—that piece of yourself that believes the message we get everyday that in order to be powerful, we must be thin and beautiful.

Will

There are two sides to the will: the will of the ego and the will of the divine. The will of the ego has no boundaries or rules. It does not respect others' space. It wants what it wants when it wants it. It rarely considers the consequences of its behavior. It is driven, confrontational, and selfish. The will of the ego will feed your bad behaviors and leave you drained, because it is constantly putting you in situations that trigger your fight-or-flight response. The will of the ego is not concerned about your well-being, preferring quick gratification, which is where most bad habits and addictions come from. The power of the ego will not surrender until it has hit bottom and recognizes it is losing, when you are totally out of control, deeply wounded, and unable to function. At this point, the ego becomes scared of losing its host—your body and mind.

This is why you cannot will your way through healing addiction. You may try to convince yourself by saying, "I can do this," yet you still keep going back to the old habits time and time again. It is like trying to lose that same ten pounds over and over. You lose it, but somehow it keeps creeping back. It is not only in your mind; this addiction is also stored in your cellular makeup. Your issues are in your tissues (and we'll discuss this more in the physical body chapter).

Although the abuse may be in the past, victims play and replay old psychological "tapes" and react mentally, emotionally, and behaviorally to events that are no longer present. Addicts become disconnected from their natural wisdom. They hear only the call of the addiction and react to it, forgetting their power of choice. They have lost their inner voice, intuition, and instinct.

Divine will works differently. It is a higher force, a knowledgeable inner feeling that arises when the mind and heart collaborate and make a final decision based on what is going on the present moment. It does not fear the inner critic of the ego.

One night I awoke from an intense dream. Spirit had been talking to me in my dream world. All of my senses were heightened. I could see, hear, and feel what Spirit wanted of me. It was so strong and clear, but it was also crazy. I wrote down everything I remembered, and the result was Boot Camp for Goddesses Level 2. I got the message that there was more information I needed to teach. This boot camp takes place in the middle of the wilderness. We live in tipis with no external distractions—no phones, no cars, no electricity. I shared my vision with my partner at the time. He thought I was nuts. I drew the vision on paper and posted it near my desk so I would see it every day. I asked Spirit to guide me and said, "If this is what I am supposed to be doing, then I will do it." I was that willful and strong about making it happen. I called my medicine woman friend, Mariam, and told her my dream. She told me that she could make the tipis. And now Boot Camp 2 is six years old. Build it and they will come. I named the new retreat Boot Camp 2: Power and Purpose.

Boot Camp 1: The Awakening helps women open to Spirit and redefine fitness, beauty, and power. Boot Camp 2 asks graduates of Boot Camp 1, now that you have this information, what are you going to do with it? What is the purpose of power if you do not use it? You may know something intellectually, but that does not mean you are living it.

This new boot camp manifested in a very short period of time, with no drama or chaos. You can easily manifest what you desire, require, and deserve if it is in alignment with your divine purpose. The energy of the universe starts to support you because you not only listen to your higher self, you follow through on the information you receive from Spirit. You have a balance between divine will and physical will. You sense it, you know it, you feel it; now you must follow through with it.

The will of the ego uses the words *want* and *need*. These are words of a victim. They exist in the future: "Someday, I want to ..." Not very powerful.

The divine will says, "I desire, require, and deserve." It is right now, in the moment: "I desire, require, and deserve a loving and healthy partner." "I desire, require, and deserve to vacation on a Florida beach this winter." You can even feel the difference and power of the words when you say them.

The higher self knows your worth and says, "I am worthy of what I desire, require, and deserve." The ego self does not. It may get there, but it probably will not enjoy the ride or experience while it is there. It is like that person in your life who is never happy, no matter what nice developments are occurring in his or her life.

The next time you share your dream with someone and they say you are crazy, are you going to allow the ego mind to be fed by that fear, or will you listen to your divine will and not care what others think?

The ego will can manifest many things, but they do not spring from a place of clarity. They most likely come through force, manipulation, and chaos, and generate bad karma in the long run. This is why you see politicians, CEOs, and others with a false sense of power fall in a dramatic way. Their willpower was misused, and eventually it caught up with them, and they lost their money, a loved one, or their health.

The divine will comes from a place of integrity and openness. It takes the time to stop, look, listen, and feel how your actions will affect you and others.

Itty-bitty Shitty Committee

I call the inner critic of the ego mind the itty-bitty shitty committee: our inner demons creating our outer world of self-betrayal and self-destruction. It truly is a committee because there are many voices at play, but they all subscribe to one belief—that you are not worthy.

The itty-bitty shitty committee is run just like a real company. There is a CEO, a vice president, a secretary, mailroom staff, and many other employees that continually ask if you really think you are worthy. Should we believe and invest in you? Are you productive for us, and do you do what we want when we want?

Visualize that you are in a beautiful Fortune 500 conference room in New York City. All the furnishings are exquisite, and there is a huge bay window overlooking Central Park. You can sense something big is coming. You have butterflies in your stomach as you wait for the CEO and staff to enter the room for your meeting.

The door opens, and like a SWAT team, the members enter the room and almost run you over in their race to take their seats. You immediately see that the members are horribly out of date—their clothes, hair, and style is stuck in a time warp. Your mind is trying to determine if what you're seeing is real or not. You take in information as a computer downloads data. You see that some people are older than others. The CEO is wearing an old polyester tie with a huge knot, a plaid suit that is so outdated it looks like one of Rodney Dangerfield's golf outfits, and he has hair growing out of his nose and eyebrows that could sweep the sidewalks of Wall Street. He is at the end of the table, standing, while all his employees are sitting, awaiting his next words as if they were the words of God.

What is going on here, you ask yourself. How this can be happening? You feel trapped in a bad dream, and the reality is, at that moment, you are. And who are you in this picture? A potential employee at an interview, waiting to see if you are worthy of their time and energy?

When you can see that your belief systems are outdated and harmful, you can heal. When you can envision the itty-bitty shitty committee in your mind and dissect them, you can turn down the volume on the ego and allow your higher self to come forward. In order to do this, you must be able to stop, look, listen, and feel if this belief system is helping you or hurting you. Ask yourself: does this take me closer to my authentic self or further away? Again and again and again, you must learn to keep your awareness in your body and alert to when your ego self is in control.

This visualization can really help shut up your itty-bitty shitty committee. The CEO represents your ego. The vice president and other employees are the old patterns, thoughts, and belief systems that follow and feed the CEO's power. Some belief systems are old and outdated, yet you can see that you have never really let them go. Some employees have more rank, just as some of our belief systems are stronger than others. From the vice president down to the mailroom operator, everyone has a job to do to keep the CEO in power. The secretary keeps track of your old past hurts and pain. The marketer feeds your doubt by continually asking, will the ego believe this or not? The coworker who constantly gossips creates judgment in your mind, and the mailroom clerk weeds out all the healthy thoughts to constantly create chaos and stop you from moving up the ladder to your higher self.

If you can see this visualization as an opportunity to reprogram your mind, it truly can be as easy as flipping a switch to shed light on the matter. You can change your perception like flipping a coin. If how you think determines how you feel, how you feel determines how you behave, and how you behave determines how you act, why can't you use the power of your imagination to create a new reality that is healing instead of self-defeating?

The next time the itty-bitty shitty committee comes knocking, envision this: you called this meeting through a memo that says, "All belief systems, please show up for a meeting. I have a new belief system I would like to introduce." You enter the conference room, waiting for the ego all its supporting belief systems to show up. They are surprised that you look radiant, ready to introduce your new belief system.

The CEO enters the room all blown up like a blowfish and ready to attack you with his darts of shame, guilt, and unworthiness. At first, you feel the fear in your belly, but you breathe into it, pray, and ask God for support, and hold your feet and body firm to the earth like a mountain. You know your new values, morals, and purpose. You know that light exists within you. And you know that now it is time to take action and turn it on full force because you will no longer hurt yourself.

The CEO realizes you are not moving and calls on the vice president to remove you. You rebel and tell him he is fired. Everyone senses your newfound strength and realizes you know they are only an illusion. You tell them, "If I created you, I can also let you go." With all your fire climbing up your spine, filling you with passion, compassion, anger, and pain, you voice your truth: "I am worthy, and I will no longer accept this behavior. You are all fired," you say. And miraculously, all the committee members leave without a fight. The power of self-love is more powerful than self-doubt. You are no longer handcuffed by their lies. You have learned the power of silence, the higher self's closest ally. You now know how to create your own destiny.

You always had this much power over the itty-bitty shitty committee. You just forgot. When did you give it up? Why? After all, you are the main stockholder in the company.

You then proceed to hire new employees—people who support your growth, your purpose, and your dreams. It could be a new partner, a new friend, or the spirit guides that you always knew existed but you shut them out because the ego mind doubted. The only people you invite to join your company are people who love you as you love yourself.

Your pain will always show you what you need to look at. It reminds you to be in your body—to stop, look, listen, and feel what needs to be healed. You can either try to numb the pain or go into the pain. When you recognize this simple fact, you can create change and write a new story for yourself.

Don't you get sick of hearing the itty-bitty shitty committee in your mind? When you allow the committee to be heard, you assume the role of victim to your past experiences and become what you fear the most: unloved and unworthy. Do you really want the itty-bitty shitty committee to have that much power over your mind and your future?

I got so tired of hearing myself talk and tell the same story, I knew I had to take action and create a new story. In order to do that, I had to release what was no longer of service to me to create new space in my mind, heart, and body. I find most women want new things, but they aren't willing to give up the old to make space for them. How can you expect to grow new things if you are not willing to weed? You have to unclog your toxic thoughts in order to start with a healthy mental body. This is the new tool every woman walks away with at Boot Camp for Goddesses. Realizing that no one ever taught them how to face their pain and reclaim, restore, and rejoice in their feminine essence, they become empowered by the understanding that they are not crazy and can be in control of their destiny.

A Healthy Mental Body

To tap into the mental body's resources, you must understand that finding balance within is necessary for growth and happiness as a human and a spiritual being. A healthy mental body knows that balance is the key to internal and external power, and that awareness is only useful if it points toward internal or external action. It does not need to manipulate anyone or anything in order to survive. It knows that Spirit will provide everything, as long you are open and receptive to hearing the call of your higher self. It knows that stillness, silence, and reflection are ways to connect to this inner voice, and it creates the space to do it daily. The mental body knows how to check in and be accountable for its words, behavior, and actions. It understands from the core that thoughts turn into matter.

Qualities OF A HEALTHY MENTAL BODY

Harmonious, clear-intentioned, focused, able to concentrate, calm, serene, receptive, observant, disciplined, nonjudgmental, noncritical, intuitive, wise, intelligent, still, silent, positive, in tune with divine will, centered, internal, quiet, peaceful, happy

A healthy mental body respects, understands, and follows the basic law of energy: it knows that thoughts have energy and that how you think determines how you feel, how you feel determines how you behave, and how you behave determines what you create.

A healthy mind no longer creates judgment or separation. It understands that everything is connected—yin and yang, male and female, healthy and unhealthy. It understands the power of choice and the consequences that follow. A healthy mental body does not separate good and bad or light and dark—it knows that everything is made from the same source, just vibrating at different frequencies. The mental body recognizes that people, thoughts, or ideas that exist at lower frequencies are still are made up of Spirit and light; they just forgot how to shine on their own and need to feed off others' energy.

The mental body knows how to flow with energy of thought without being used by it. A healthy mental body does not put itself above or below any of the other bodies or anyone else, and it always knows what is healthy for it at any given moment.

When balanced, the mental body knows how turn off the chatter from the outside world and uses the will of the divine to guide and keep you on your divine path. It does not fear what people will think. Instead, it asks, "Am I doing the right thing for myself and all involved?" A healthy mental body does not fear truth. It knows that everything comes from the void of the universe, a place of silence and stillness where answers are found and things are created. It knows to always ask if each thought and experience is taking you deeper into your core and closer to your higher self or taking you further away. A healthy mental body is able to recognize unhealthy thoughts—such as illusion, fear, and self-sabotage—generated by the ego mind that seek to stop you from feeling and being worthy of love.

A healthy mental body knows there is a sacred place inside of us all where everything is still; a place where questions are asked and answers are found. Stillness is the space between heartbeats. Silence is the pause between breaths. When you go deeper into the practice of stillness and silence, as discussed in the spiritual body chapter, you can go deeper into mastering your mind. Being able to stop, look, listen, and feel plays an important role in keeping the mental body healthy. In this process, the mind is able to hear the inner voice of your intuition. It is also able to create its vision. Being silent enables the mental body to align with the divine will. The receptivity of the spiritual body and the focus, concentration, and discipline of the mental body set the course for the emotional and physical bodies to follow. And when all four bodies are aligned, you can bring your divine purpose and your dreams to life. When you learn to fully trust your intuition without doubt or fear, you uncover and balance your power internally and externally. As you start working with the spiritual body, then the mental body on down, you start the process of finding your fragmented pieces and becoming a whole and holy person again. When you truly grasp that your thoughts determine your reality, it changes your perspective on all things within you and surrounding you.

A healthy mental body gives you the courage to go inward and express your thoughts outwardly. You are able to discern what is true and what is not for yourself. You say what you mean and mean what you say. With a healthy mental body, you are able to hear your inner voice and listen to your body's intelligence. You can feel with your mind and think with your heart about what your body is telling you and how to respect this inner knowing. You no longer deny this wisdom but search deeper into it, knowing that it is a gift from God.

A healthy mind listens to the feelings of the heart and will not deny what the heart wants to feel and express—helpful and inspiring thoughts that inform your core values and build strong and healthy belief systems. When your mental body is healthy, you do not need to wear masks. You know who you are and are proud of it. You accept all parts of yourself. You are in tune with your ancestors and know those who walked before you. You do not judge them; you are proud of them, because you know that they are you and you are them. You understand that love is more than just an emotion; it is a powerful force capable of healing yourself and others, and it resides within you just waiting to be unleashed.

You know your own personal space and your boundaries—where you end and another begins. You do not take things personally but are able to distinguish whether what you hear is true for you or not. You can speak your truth no matter the consequences, because you know how someone else perceives your words is not your responsibility as long as you speak from your own spiritual integrity.

You understand that silence and stillness are nourishment for your mind and spirit, and reflection is a time for you to tap into your true beauty so that you can shine internally and externally. You no longer react but act, creating your own destiny instead of allowing your environment to do it for you. You will never fall victim again.

In a healthy mental body, the ego and inner critic still exist, but they support the intuition by being quiet and still instead of drowning it out or turning it off altogether.

If you hear your intuition and do not follow it, your ego will not shame you or blame you for things going wrong. It will simply ask why you chose not to listen and to resist. A healthy ego knows its place.

An Unhealthy Mental Body

When the mind is not able to be still and silent, it creates a buildup of thoughts and energy that results in irritability and nervous energy. This puts a lot of tension on the nervous system and keeps the physical body in a constant state of fight-or-flight. Over time, this state can pave the way for depression, ADD, weight gain, hormone imbalances, and heart palpitations to develop.

An unhealthy mental body does not listen to your inner voice or recognize the body's intelligence. It looks for answers outside itself, creating a fogginess in the mind. When the mental body is not guided by the higher self, it doesn't know what direction to go in and allows outside influences to control its destiny. It only responds to doubt and fear and moves away from pain. It will keep you overstriving or lifeless, both of which have numbing effects over time. The senses also become dull and can no longer touch, taste, smell, hear, and see Spirit within them and surrounding them. They lose their connection to nature, which is calming and restores breathing to naturally full levels. (This is why people who are depressed do not like to go outside.)

Qualities
OF AN UNHEALTHY MENTAL BODY

Disharmonious, overreactive, controlling, nervous, egotistical, overanalytical, judgmental, critical, dramatic, chaotic, restless, foolish, arrogant, narcissistic

An unhealthy mental body creates suffering and more pain by making the situation worse than it is or by going into total denial. It is either stuck in the past or reaching into the future—it is never in the present moment. It fears stillness and silence, because it fears the truth. It is by turns willful and lazy, forceful and victimized, overenergized and underenergized—all extremes that serve to keep the mind from focusing on anything but the truth.

An unhealthy mental body resists taking the time to reflect, because it knows it will have to deal with thoughts and feelings that might be painful. "The mind will not allow what the heart wants to feel" is the mantra of the unhealthy mental body. This is how the mental body and emotional body weave together in an unhealthy way.

Belief systems created by an unhealthy mind separate the higher self from Spirit. An imbalanced mental body does not believe in faith, hope, or trust. Rather, it is driven by the practical and rational mind. It always wants to see proof.

An unhealthy mind fears intimacy and won't allow you to look people in the eyes, either because it does not feel worthy, fears confrontation, or wants to stay hidden. It creates separation of good and evil and only sees things in extremes. The constant stress of up/down wreaks havoc on the mind and nervous system and drowns out intuition and body intelligence, breeding either overconfidence or a constant fearfulness.

Meditation is torture for the unhealthy mental body because it resists sitting still and observing. Even a quiet walk can be uncomfortable if your mental body is out of balance—your mind would rather talk and fill the silence than be quiet enough to listen. The mind's selfishness will cause you to stay removed from the people around you and to ignore boundaries between yourself and others.

The unhealthy mental body has an unhealthy ego. It does not support the intuition; it shuts it down. It also wears many masks because it has a false sense of self. After all, the imbalanced mental body is never true to itself—how could it show its true self to others? It keeps itself busy by constantly comparing itself to others and becoming obsessed with keeping score.

In our culture, men tend to have overdeveloped mental bodies—a means of survival in the cold, cruel business world. Their ego is centered around themselves and their accomplishments. Women are typically the opposite (though this is changing as more women enter the work force). A woman tends to focus more on the needs of her family than herself. Mothers hold their children at the center of their world. The point of reference for their ego is external (their children); thus they appear egoless, or selfless. All the mother's thoughts, feelings, and identity are invested in another.

When you fear the parts of yourself that you do not like, you create separation, which results in judgment, which separates us from the source. As a result, you do not feel worthy of love—self-love or otherwise. When you cannot love yourself, you look to people and things outside yourself to make you feel worthy. It leads to addiction, depression, codependence, and mental illness.

$\mathcal{A}$N UNHEALTHY MENTAL BODY

A medical perspective from Jeff Migdow, M.D.

I FIND IN my work that imbalances in the mental body (ruled by the air element) are often due to overstimulation. Think of our grade-school education: so much emphasis is put on mental capabilities and hardly any on physical development and health, emotional understanding and balance, and spiritual connection. The institution food is unhealthy, most states have cut gym class down to once or twice a week, expression of emotion is suppressed, and there is no training for connecting to our inner self, intuition, or Spirit. Thus, most of us feel a constant mental tension from an early age.

The result of this overstimulation is anxiety, insomnia, a lack of spiritual connection, a tendency to always be in the past or the future, emotional upset such as anger and impatience, and the stress-related diseases of headache, backache, irritable bowel syndrome, gastric reflux from overeating and eating too quickly, and heart palpitations, among others. It's as if there were a strong wind constantly blowing through our system, overactivating our mind, putting stress on all parts of our system, and perpetually blowing us off-course.

If we can utilize tools to help calm and clear the mental body, we gain relaxation, calm, mental clarity, focus, a deeper connection to our intuition, emotional balance, and physical relaxation. Simply practicing relaxation breathing a few minutes an hour with a longer relaxation at the end of the day can put us on the road to rebalancing and calming our mental body.

Disease of the Mental Body: A Case Study

An elderly female patient of mine, whom I have seen on and off for years, is chronically experiencing heart palpitations and bowel pains and spasms. When she has gotten to the point where the palpitations are keeping her awake at night and/or her bowel spasms have progressed into painful bowel distress, she sees me to get back on track.

Invariably, she explains that the stresses of life have caught up to her again, and she needs help with her physical symptoms. She has totally lost touch with the fact that her mental body has gone out of whack. As we begin to talk, I remind her that it's not the actual stresses but her mental reaction to them that is the problem—that it's her mind's tendency to get afraid and then project into the future that throws her off-course.

I work with her to remind her that if she can stay present, she can connect to her intuition and find solutions to her problems that solve them much more deeply and easily than the piecemeal bandage solutions of her mind. We go over the tools that help calm her mind down and bring it back to the present, including taking time to do slow, deep breathing often during the day, stretching the tension out of her body, and slowing down. Every time, she reports that when she remembers to slow down, she becomes more efficient in performing her daily tasks and she actually gains time, which she can use to breathe and stretch more. Finally, what works best for her is taking time each night to play soothing music and repeat affirmations that she has the ability to be present in her life.

Within four weeks of her initial appointment, she's back on track, and the effects generally last for one to two years. She says she uses me to help remind her of what she needs to do for herself. This is an important point. Although we do have all the answers within us, in our hectic, overstimulated life, we can lose touch with our inner knowing and forget the tools we have at our disposal. An important tool, then, is to have people in our life, privately or professionally, that we can call on when we need reminders and support. I always have at least three people in my life whom I can call on when I feel my connection to what works for me is slipping away. This human support is extremely powerful and helpful—it gets me back on course, reminds my friend to also do the things that make him or her feel better, and strengthens our connection to each other. I also believe it helps raise the vibration of humanity in general.

Self-Test to Discover the Current State of Your Mental Body

The following questionnaire is designed to enable you to find your strengths and weaknesses in the mental body. It is also beneficial for strengthening self-awareness, which is key in being able to objectively see yourself clearly and from there be able to create more openness, strength, and balance in your life.

Take time for each question, and answer in a way that feels truthful to you. If you have areas where you feel like you aren't being honest, know that these are the places in which you tend to fool yourself. Usually these are the areas that need the most work.

Give yourself 5 points for *always*, 4 for *often*, 3 for *sometimes*, 2 for *occasionally*, and 1 for *never*. Then add up your totals for each body to get the grand total. This will help you objectively see where you stand in this body. As you move through this book and take the tests for the other bodies, compare the totals to see where your imbalances lie. We suggest you redo each of these questionnaires every one to two months to check your progress and give you time to reflect.

Questions	
Key: always (5 points), often (4), sometimes (3), occasionally (2), never (1)	
1. I use my mental creativity to support my health and well-being.	4
2. I am generally relaxed and unworried.	3
3. I take time to relax daily.	2
4. My communications are open and harmonious.	3

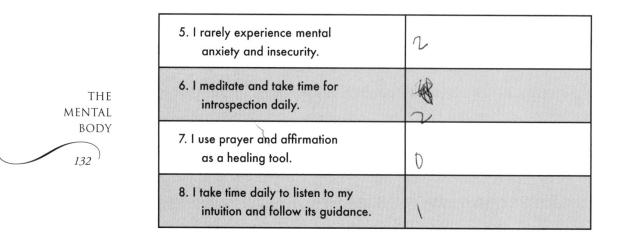

5. I rarely experience mental anxiety and insecurity.	2
6. I meditate and take time for introspection daily.	2
7. I use prayer and affirmation as a healing tool.	0
8. I take time daily to listen to my intuition and follow its guidance.	1

Tally your score by adding up the points that correspond to each of your answers, and jot it down in a notebook or journal. Although 40 is a perfect score, where you fall on the scale today is not as important as seeing your scores improve over time, both numerically and in relation to your other bodies (you don't want one score to be off the charts with others far behind, for example). As you test all four bodies, you'll begin to see how you can bring more balance to your entire being. If, for example, you scored a 36 on your spiritual body fitness and later realize that your physical body fitness is only a 14, you can use that information to bring those numbers onto a more equal plane, perhaps by meditating less and working out more.

Strengthening the Mental Body

Rebuilding the mental body establishes clarity and sanity. When the mind is still, the heart can open, and you can access the body's natural and holistic intelligence to grow (physically), learn (mentally), love (emotionally), and evolve (spiritually). In order to radiate without, you must create balance within—or, as I often say at boot camp, you have to slow down to catch up. These exercises will help you get quiet and sit still so that you can weed out toxic thoughts, focus on the present moment, and act according to your inborn intelligence and intuition. They work whether you need clarity or calm stimulation, or both.

AN INSIDE-OUT WORKOUT
FOR THE MENTAL BODY

The following tools and exercises are practices to focus and open the mental body. I call them mental push-ups, as they strengthen all the muscles of the mental body, connect you to your native wisdom, and strengthen your truth.

Reflection

As you learned earlier, you have 50,000 thoughts a day, with the negative far outweighing the positive. Meditating creates space between your thoughts so you can hear your own inner voice. When you can learn the discipline of silence and stillness of the mind, you can then identify and pull the weeds that take up too much space in your mind. You can ask yourself, "Is this thought worthy of my time and energy? Is it my thought or was it projected on me by someone else? Is it true for me? Does this thought illuminate or support what I desire, require, and deserve?" And most importantly, "Do I have space for this thought in my body and my life?"

Because I believe you can never hear it enough: *how you think determines how you feel, how you feel determines how you behave, and how you behave determines what you create.* And in order to shut down your mental doubting and nagging, you must first create space in the mind. Practicing the discipline of silence and stillness gives you the opportunity to stop, look, listen, and feel the thoughts in your mind and get rid of what doesn't serve you, thereby creating space. When you learn how to turn down the volume on your negative thoughts, your inner voice can be heard, and you can get a clearer picture of what it is that you truly desire, require, and deserve.

*You gain strength, courage and confidence
from every experience by which you really stop
to look fear in the face. You are able to say
to yourself, "I lived through this horror.
I can take the next thing that comes along."*
—ELEANOR ROOSEVELT

You then move to the next level of being able to reflect on the past, present, and future. You can look back at your past like looking into an archive and determine what worked and what did not; this is how you develop wisdom. When you can reflect, you can see yourself with deep respect and love. But you must create the space in your life to hear your inner voice so that you can set your direction to be moving toward it.

When you reflect, you can see yourself in the big picture and see how others are just mirrors of your present state. You no longer assign blame and assume the role of victim. You look at each situation to see what it has to show you or teach you instead of what it is doing to you.

Similar to the soul-searching exercise I discussed in the spiritual body chapter, try staring into Mother Nature's eyes. Sit under a tree, on a mountain, or in your garden and gaze at a natural object—a tree, a plant, a rock, or a geological formation—and feel its essence as yours. You will learn how every rock, tree, and mountain has a face and spirit, just as you do. When you are able to release your fears and doubts, you become one with this object and its beauty instead of experiencing it as an entity separate from yourself.

Benefits:

- Teaches stillness.

- Promotes silence.

- Improves focus.

Labyrinth

The labyrinth is one of the oldest contemplative and transformational tools known to humankind, dating back to AD 500. Labyrinths have been used by the Hopi Navajos, Anasazi Indians, and ancient Greeks, Romans, French, Syrians, Spanish, North Africans, and Russians. There is a labyrinth on the floor of the French cathedral Notre-Dame de Chartres; people would walk on their knees through the labyrinth while chanting the rosary.

In a labyrinth, there is only one route to the center and back again (unlike a maze, which is filled with dead-ends). No matter where you are in a labyrinth, you can always see the center. The labyrinth ritual and practice will lead you not only to the center of the labyrinth itself but also to the center of yourself. Walking a labyrinth is a meditative and symbolic discipline of setting one foot in front of the other. It is very reflective exercise, helping you observe how you walk through your journey of life—fast, slow, or hesitating; in a straight line or meandering.

Walking a labyrinth helps you tap into your inborn intelligence. The spiral is the symbol of the labyrinth as well as the winding strands of DNA where our native wisdom resides. The spiral represents the winding journey of birth, death, and rebirth. It is a ritual that allows you to walk with Spirit.

When building my own labyrinth in the mountains of Colorado, I recognized the similarities between the rainbow and the labyrinth. Both structures are a gateway to help the human spirit touch Spirit itself. The Bible declares the rainbow a covenant between Earth and God. The classical labyrinth is the shape of a rainbow with seven arches. The seven colors of the rainbow are also the seven colors of the chakras. The seven arches of the labyrinth are also similar to the seven chakras, since chakras are wheels of energy spinning in a spiraling motion. (There are also seven temples on the Inca trail leading up to Machu Picchu. Each temple helps you awaken to the healing power within you and surrounding you.)

Whether you walk a labyrinth on foot or in your mind, you will always find the center, *your* center, when you walk toward the light, truth, and wholeness of the matter. This is where transformation is found.

Benefits:

- Brings balance to the right and left hemispheres of the brain as well as your thoughts and emotions.

- Opens you to your own intuition and invites Spirit to guide you on your journey.

- Enables you to listen to your own voice and walk your own path with confidence and surrender.

Tratak

Tratak, or steady gazing, is an excellent concentration exercise. It involves alternately gazing at an object or point without blinking, then closing your eyes and visualizing the object in your mind's eye. The practice steadies the wandering mind and concentrates the attention, leading you to focus with pinpoint accuracy. Wherever the eyes go, the mind follows.

1. Place an object—such as a burning candle, a shell, or a pinecone—at eye level, three feet away from you.

2. Spend a few moments concentrating on the sound of your breath, and wait until your breathing has settled into a deeper, slower rhythm.

3. Begin gazing at the object without blinking. Don't stare or gaze vacantly—look steadily, without straining.

4. After about a minute, close your eyes, keeping your inner gaze steady, and visualize the object in your mind's eye—the third eye, where your intuition lives.

5. When the after-image vanishes, open your eyes and repeat.

Benefits:

- Focuses and steadies the mind.

- Promotes concentration and focus.

- Allows the mind to take on the qualities of what it is focusing on—a tree brings peacefulness and strength, while water brings calmness and flow, for example.

- Teaches you how to stay in the present moment.

- Strengthens your ability to see and read energy.

- Creates space in the mind, lowering the number of thoughts in a day.

- Teaches the ego to be silent and still.

- Strengthens your ability to hear your inner voice.

- Balances the left and right hemispheres of the brain.

- Strengthens pituitary and pineal glands, bringing balance to hormones.

Yantras

Yantra is a Sanskrit word derived from the root *yam*, which means "to control, subdue, restrain, curb, or check." A yantra is a diagram or drawing designed to help control the mind and often contains squares, triangles, flowers, and circles. The Shri Yantra is one of the most famous and ancient yantras; it is an arrangement of nine triangles with five downward-pointing triangles, representing the female forces of the universe, and four upward-pointing triangles, representing the male forces.

Yantras come from the Tantric tradition, which is more than 2,000 years old. A yantra is the equivalent of the Buddhist mandala. To do this exercise, use the illustrations on the following page for the object, and follow the same instructions as for tratak.

1. Place an object—in this case, any of the four yantras on the following page—at eye level, three feet away from you.

2. Spend a few moments concentrating on the sound of your breath, and wait until your breathing has settled into a deeper, slower rhythm.

3. Begin gazing at the yantra without blinking. Don't stare or gaze vacantly—look steadily, without straining.

4. After about a minute, close your eyes, keeping your inner gaze steady, and visualize the yantra in your mind's eye—the third eye, where your intuition lives.

5. When the after-image vanishes, open your eyes and repeat.

Benefits:
- Improves ability to visualize.
- Builds concentration.
- Opens the mind to Spirit.
- Promotes relaxation.

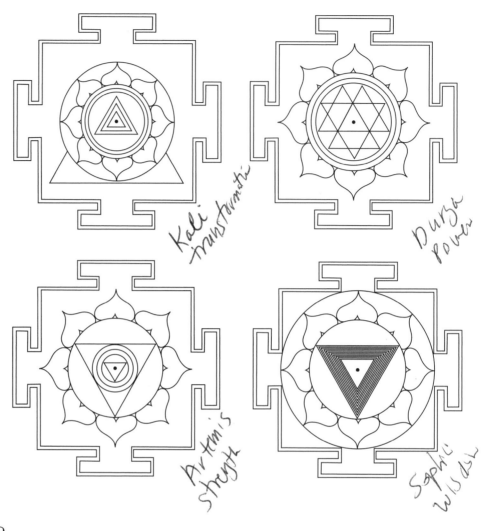

Kali transformation

Durga power

Artemis strength

Sophia wisdom

𝒴*antras, clockwise from top left: Kali, the goddess of transformation (root chakra; by overcoming all fears, especially the fear of death, deep spiritual transformation is possible); Durga, the goddess of power (the sexual chakra; gives great powers to her devotees by establishing a powerful connection to the self and the energy of the universe to win all battles and overcome all adversities); Artemis, warrior goddess (the goddess of strength, core solar plexus chakra; cultivates her inner strength to overcome obstacles within and surrounding her, setting boundaries to allow her kundalini to flow); and Sophia, the goddess of wisdom and intuition (third eye chakra; cuts off the chattering mind and allows you to tap into the kundalini energy moving up).*

Aromatherapy

Essential oils are highly concentrated extracts distilled from herbs, flowers, and trees. They are the regenerative, oxygenating, and immunity-defending properties of plants. Essential oils contain vitamins, minerals, and natural antiseptics. They are to the plant what the immune and hormone systems are to the human body. When you break a leaf off an aloe plant, a liquid substance will bleed from the plant. This is the life force of the plant, just as blood is the life force of a human. A molecule of the hemoglobin in our blood has similar properties to a molecule of chlorophyll—the blood of the plant kingdom.

Since the nostrils are so close to the brain and nervous system, your sense of smell is a powerful way to affect the mental body. When inhaled, essential oils can affect every cell of the body within twenty minutes and are metabolized like other nutrients. They trigger the brain to release serotonin, leaving you with a feeling of bliss and peace of mind. They also affect the limbic system, the primitive part of the brain that controls the fight-or-flight response, causing it to release emotional issues that are stored in the body's connective tissues and the nervous system.

Because there is so much pollution today, our most primitive sense—the sense of smell—is becoming dulled, the result of which can include headaches, loss of memory, overstimulated nervous systems, Parkinson's disease, Alzheimer's disease, Lou Gehrig's disease, and multiple sclerosis. If how you think is how you feel, how you feel is how you behave, and how you behave is what you create, you must take responsibility for your environment and all that you inhale. Candles, perfumes, oils, pollution, paint, carpet—the very things that are found in our homes, offices, cities, and world—can all leach invisible toxins. And if you think you are not exposed to these invisible toxins, think again. Why do you have migraines? Why are you or your children suffering from asthma, sinus infections, irritability, or even bad dreams? Asthma is spreading like wildfire across our nation and affecting many people because of the toxins we smell and eat and the overload of stimuli in our environment. It is scary and quite frankly killing the next generation's ability to connect to Mother Earth and her most natural medicine—fresh air.

Through my own healing process I refused to take drugs, knowing they would only numb me out. I knew I needed to learn how to relax. I treated myself to a weekly massage to reprogram my nervous system. The therapist was also a professional aromatherapist who made her own essential blends from her garden. She would have me pick my own oil every time I came and would have me smell different oils to see which appealed to me the most—your body knows what it needs. I would immediately feel soothed. I could not believe the effects those essential oils had on me so quickly. My therapist would rub this oil on my body during the massage and place it on cotton balls in the head rest so I was inhaling it for about an hour and half. She also would rub it directly on my spine—the conduit of the nervous system. I would then take home the oil and every day smell this oil for a minute in each nostril several times a day. After months of repeating this exercise and treatment, I could see how my body was healing. My jaw was not as tight, and my body was more relaxed. I had no more headaches or nightmares, and I was more receptive to my environment. This was over fifteen years ago, and to this day I continue this practice. It is a huge part of my life and key to my sanity. I healed myself for the rest of my life without taking drugs to temporarily put out the fire of my discomfort.

To do this exercise, you will need the purest lavender oil you can find. Do not buy any essential oil if it is mixed with something else or if it is not in a dark bottle. The dark bottle keeps light out, because light breaks down the oil's healing properties. A good test is also to smell the oil. If you do not feel it affect your whole body like a wave running down your spine, and if it only stops at your nostrils, then you are not dealing with a pure essential oil. Again, the nose knows. When you smell an essential oil, it will stimulate your whole nervous system. It will either soothe you, give you energy, or bring up a memory stored in your cells (we'll discuss this more in the emotional body).

Healers and holy people have used essentials oils for thousands of years, yet this knowledge has been taken away from us because of the fear of witchcraft. It's time to reclaim these beautiful healing tools as our own again and put a stop to all the illness within us and surrounding us. We have to slow down to catch up and go back to our most primitive ways in order to heal—connecting to Mother Earth's wisdom, strength, compassion, and openness.

1. Holding a bottle of lavender in your left hand, sit in an erect position, head up, back straight, and heart open.

2. Place your right index finger on the right side of your nose to close off the nostril.

3. Hold the bottle of lavender oil under your left nostril and breathe in and out only through your left nostril for ten big breaths.

4. Repeat with right nostril.

Other ways to use essential oils to detoxify your space and bring peace to your mind and nervous system include:

- Place on cotton balls and use in your dryer as a natural freshener.

- Place on cotton balls to use in your car as a natural freshener, or sprinkle some on the floor of your car.

- Sprinkle on your pillow cases—pure essential oil will not stain.

- Sprinkle on natural bee honey or soy candles.

- Dab a little bit on your fingertips and rub the oil gently into your temples and under your nostrils so that you are constantly breathing it in. Be sure not to get inside your nostril, as it will burn.

- Place in your humidifier.

- I even use it with my animals; I place some under my horse's nostrils and on his temples.

Benefits:
- Soothes the nervous system.

- Relaxes, calms, and centers.

- Balances the right and left hemispheres of the brain.

- Releases serotonin into the brain.

- Reprograms the nervous system.

- Releases cellular memory in the mind and connective tissue.

Crystals

Just as essential oils have healing properties for the mind, body, and spirit, so do crystals, rocks, and minerals. The natives call rocks the ancient ones or the grandfathers. They are believed to be the oldest and wisest beings on this planet, for they make up the earth. During a sweat lodge ceremony, we pray to the stone people, our grandfathers, for their wisdom and to cleanse us of the dis-ease within us and surrounding us.

And just as essential oils are living beings, so are minerals, crystals, and rock formations. They have created some of the most beautiful places on earth, such as the Patagonia fjords, Yosemite National Park, the Grand Canyon, and many more. They are the wonders of the world that continually connect us and make us look inward to bring forth our primitive intelligence. The grandfathers remind us of how young and immature we are, how minute we are in the world, and they have the ability to heal us. Animals eat minerals and plants in order to gain the nutrients that their bodies need to survive. The same iron ore that is in the earth is in our own bloodstream and courses through our veins to keep our body strong and blood healthy. When we resonate with these elements, the resources of the earth, we strengthen our own vital forces. The next time you sit on a rock or hold a crystal, honor its life force by validating its intelligence. It was here a long time before you.

Every rock and mineral has its own personality. Each one holds a vibration, a frequency that helps us align our own personal energy to come back into balance with the earth's vibration. This internal alignment will put you back into your body and reconnect you to your energetic umbilical cord connecting you to your true mother, Mother Earth, Gaea. This is what it means and feels like to be present and grounded.

Crystals reflect and hold light that gives off healing vibrations. You will be attracted to certain stones for different reasons, depending on where your energy is at that moment. You will be drawn to hold it or place it on your body. Natives use the stones for healing their energetic field as well as diseases. They also wear certain stones as jewelry to let others know their stature in the tribe and to ward off lower frequencies.

The next time you are attracted to a rock, crystal, or mineral, pay attention to what it is telling you. You may feel the need to meditate with it, hold it for soothing, or just admire its beauty. Whatever your reason, know it is talking to you in more ways than one.

As an example, amethyst is the color purple, the color of the third eye chakra, the energy point in between our eyes. As the smell of lavender is connected to the third eye and the pineal and pituitary glands, so is the amethyst. It is a stone used in the breast-plate of the high priest and the gemstone of royalty.

When your intuition is strengthened, you will hear what the stone people have to say to you. You will resonate with their messages and heal more than you could ever imagine. Believe and you will receive the magic of the Mother Earth. Hug stones just as you would hug a tree, whether it be in your hand or as you lie on a massive stone with your heart and third eye on it. Next time you go for walk or meditate outside, see if you can take the time to reconnect to Mother Earth. If you are uncomfortable or unsure of how to do this, hang out with a young child for a day. He or she will teach you.

All my nieces come into my home to play with my drums, crystals, cards, and books—wherever their heart and intuition lead them. They know my home is a place to relax and come back to their true nature. They shoot the bow and arrow with me, sing songs, give offerings to the animals, hug trees, and connect to Mother Earth. My four-year-old niece Bella recently told me a story about the stone and tree people. She told me that when she was playing in the woods behind her yard, she wandered off by herself, away from her sisters. Then she heard the wind speaking to her to leave the place she was in and to go back to the house. On her way home, she heard the stone people also tell her she must stay on track and go home. Then she heard a tree speak to her, and she noticed the tree had strange marks on it and the bark was missing. That's when she started running and got home as quickly as possible.

I asked her to show me this place in the woods. When I saw the tree she mentioned, I noticed the scrapes and nail markings of a black bear. Any bear will mark the trees as its territory. Bella had listened to her intuition, and she was validated by Mother Earth and by me. When she shared this story, there were other, older children around. They laughed and told her she was crazy, but she did not care, for she knew she was right down to her bones. And I was there to support and validate her story. This is a story that has strengthened her connection to Mother Earth as well as her intuition and native intelligence.

Think how mountains and glaciers—all different faces of the stone people—have attracted native tribes throughout history, such Buddhist monks in the Himalayas, the Quero in the Peruvian Andes, several Native American tribes in Colorado, and the Amazons and Incas at Machu Picchu in the Andes. They all knew that the healing energy of the stone people is where the ancient wisdom of Mother Earth resides.

How to Use Crystals

1. Place crystals under your pillows and sleep with them there.

2. Hold a crystal while you meditate.

3. Put crystals near your computer to counteract the negative ions the electricity emits.

4. Place crystals on your body as you rest in corpse pose.

Benefits:

- Clears fogginess from the mind.

- Sharpens the thinking process.

- Brings a feeling of overall peace.

- Treats nervous system disorders such as insomnia, heart complications, and addiction.

- Stimulates psychic abilities and helps you integrate your spiritual lessons, keeping you on the path of divine will and connected to your higher self.

Journaling

Journaling is a wonderful tool to integrate your thoughts and feelings. It helps you vent on the page, to release what you are holding in or holding back. It is also a wonderful way to keep track of your progress and your setbacks. I found journaling was my savior after my near-death experience. Everyone thought I was losing my mind. I was so aligned with Spirit that when I opened my mouth, I could not believe what came out. I was channeling and didn't even know it. I felt like a minister giving a Sunday sermon. Journaling allowed me to speak my truth on paper and release my fears of telling my truth. It helped me develop my own personal relationship with God.

Over time, I trained my higher self to ask questions before I went to bed. I would write the question I needed an answer for, such as, *why am I having dreams about a runaway car that I cannot stop?* Your higher consciousness comes forward in the dream world, and nightmares are usually when the lower self and the higher self are in an argument. In the dream world, you can receive answers and fight your worst enemy—your lower self. I would awake with answers always between 3 and 5 AM, because when we are in REM sleep, our higher self moves to the forefront and our spirit guides give us messages.

When you are able to train your brain to have a dialog with your higher self, you can create your destiny on a whole other level. The book you hold in your hands started off as journaling.

The best part for me was when I looked back at my journals years later, I could not believe how much I had grown spiritually, mentally, emotionally, and physically. They became proof of my internal and external success.

I always keep a journal to write down my thoughts, whether it is just brief words here and there or long hours of writing. While you drive, your mind automatically goes into reflection if you do not have the music blaring. Some of my best ideas come in the car or on the plane.

Benefits:

- Focuses the mind on experiences of the day.
- Allows the mind to learn from experience.
- Provides an avenue to integrate the day's experiences.
- Provides a mental and emotional release.
- Provides a source for channeling.

Archery

As you get still and take aim, bow, arrow, goal, and ego all melt into one another. The need to separate has gone. The bow and arrow is both a weapon for protection and a tool used to obtain food. Practical, it is easy to carry, does not make loud noises that could scare prey, and uses flint and wood, resources you can find anywhere in nature.

The bow requires strength to pull, flexibility to bend, and wisdom to know when to let go. Practicing archery is a meditative yet physical art of balance. It cultivates a calm yet focused mind, strong yet flexible body, and an open heart yet grounded body.

Even as you do bow pose in yoga, these are the questions you must ask yourself: Do I know when to let go? What is my target in life? Can I remain focused, or do I allow outside chatter to distract me?

Throughout history, native tribes, including the Amazon women warriors, used the bow as a life-sustaining tool. The Amazon women received their name from the Spanish army. They were known for their mastery of archery and their fierce fighting tactics. *Amazon* means "one-breasted"—in Greek, *mazos* means "breast," and *a* means "without." The myth is that the Amazon women cut off one breast to better shoot the bow and arrow. In Armenia, Amazon means moon-women, in Persia it means warrior, in Libya a free or noble person. All of these definitions describe the fiercest tribe of warriors in history.

The bow is believed to have been invented between 8000 and 9000 BC. Arrowheads have been found that date back 50,000 years ago. More recently, women studied archery while men played golf—women competed in the 1908 Olympics with longbows.

Archery is also a major practice of Zen Buddhism. Zen archery master Awa Kenzo teaches, "In Zen archery, art becomes artless, shooting becomes not-shooting, and the archer becomes the target."

I have been practicing archery and hunting with my bow since 2000. It is a feeling of power when you hear the arrow release, see it spiraling through the air, and hear the *bang* as it hits the target. There's a hormone surge, a feeling of "Yes! I am a warrior." The adrenaline rush gets your blood pumping and heart beating.

When I teach archery to women, it is such a metaphor. Before we start, they are unable to focus, stay on course, pull the bow back, open their heart, or stay grounded in their body. It's a reflection that they are not ready to own their power mentally or physically. They pull back, and the arrow will drop. And it is amazing to see how their anger can help them overcome when they learn how to focus it. It is primal and quite sexy to own all that power. They feel the rush up their spine and are soon begging for more. "Let me at it," they say, not aware of how powerful this practice can be—they now have a target for all their pent-up emotions, and the relief they feel when they let go is major. At the same time, they are owning their power—physically strong, mentally focused, emotionally in tune, and spiritually connected.

Next time you need a sport for yourself or your daughter, try archery. You can even do it in your back yard. My nieces were able to do it from as early as age three.

Benefits:
- Creates one-pointed focus.
- Helps you let go of expectations.
- Calms the mind.

- Fosters discipline.

- Strengthens the upper back, chest, and arms.

- Expresses anger or any pent-up emotions in a healthy way.

- Helps you stay in alignment with your goals and dreams.

BREATHING FOR THE MENTAL BODY

Air Breath/Alternate Nostril Breath
Sanskrit name: Nadi Breath

Air breath is the element of air, wind, and thoughts. It is the breath of relaxation and concentration.

1. Start in a seated or kneeling position with your spine erect.

2. Place your right hand in front of your face with the palm facing you.

3. Close your right nostril with your right thumb and inhale through your left nostril for the count of four.

4. Close the left nostril with your right ring finger and forcefully exhale out of the right nostril. Then inhale for the count of four in the same nostril.

5. Close off the right nostril with your right thumb and exhale through your left nostril. Repeat, alternating nostrils. Inhale for the count of four and exhale for the count of eight.

Continue for 3–5 minutes and work up to fifteen minutes throughout your day.

Benefits:
- Improves the balance between the left and right hemispheres of the brain.

- Releases serotonin into the brain, helpful with addictive habits and hormone harmony.

- Creates balance of opposing energies such as yin/yang, female/male, and intuition/intellect.

- Restores balance to the nervous system and helps ease anxiety and nervous system illnesses such as Parkinson's and MS.

- Prevents migraine headaches and relieves migraines.

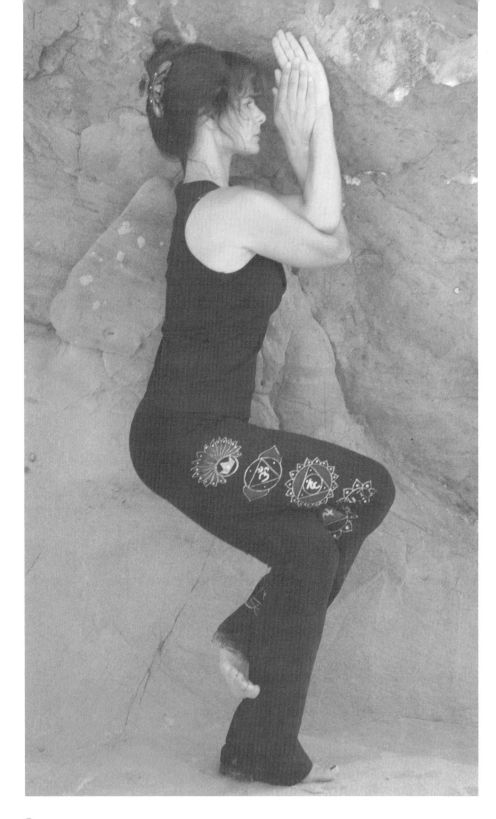

 *Eagle pose*

YOGA POSES FOR THE MENTAL BODY

Yoga is the science and practice of self: self-awareness, self-acceptance, and self-love. Each posture will reflect your weaknesses and strengths. Are you able to go into pain or do you run from pain? Breathe, have patience, and know that yoga is not about being flexible but being in the present moment so that you can stop, look, listen, and feel what is going on within. It is about intention, not perfection. The physical body will always benefit from what you do internally first and work its way out to the external.

Eagle Pose/Vision
Sanskrit Name: Garudasana

The divine bird, the eagle, is a powerful symbol. Its exquisite vision leads to enlightenment. This divine bird soars majestically above the earth, seeing all. Connect your soul to the eagle and fly majestically toward enlightenment. The eagle says, "I see clearly; I fly to freedom on the strength of my inner being." Are you free to fly?

Entry and Holding Posture

1. Start by standing tall with integrity, feet firmly connected to the ground, heart open, head facing up toward the sky. Bend your knees slightly and lift your left foot up while balancing on your right foot, with all four corners of your foot in contact with ground.

2. Cross your left thigh over the right. Point your left toes toward the ground, and hook the top of the foot behind the lower right calf. Keep balancing on the right foot.

3. Standing firm in your right leg, press the sole of your foot into the floor and squeeze your inner thighs together.

4. Bending deeper into the standing leg, bring your pelvis into an upright, neutral position as much as possible.

5. Bring your arms out to the sides to open the chest, then cross the left elbow over the right in front of the body and interlace the arms, working toward a position with the palms of the hands pressed together and the elbows lifted.

6. Relax your shoulders and draw the shoulder blades down the back, squeezing your elbows and hands together as you press the outer borders of the shoulders away from each other. Your back, neck, and head should remain straight. Continue balancing by stabilizing your right foot.

7. Feel all the cells of your being coming into alignment as they resonate with life source energy. Notice your spiral of energy coming through the earth and rising up to the third eye, instilling centeredness, enlightenment, and clarity and connecting you from earth to heaven.

8. Release and rest in the harmony of every cell being attuned to the spiral blueprint of life.

Repeat on opposite side, crossing the left leg over the right and left arm over the right. Hold up to 15–30 seconds each side—about five big breaths only through the nostrils.

Benefits and Systems Being Treated, Challenged, and Healed:

- Increases circulation in joints.

- Improves digestion and elimination.

- Rejuvenates circulatory system.

- Tones the pulmonary and nervous systems, digestive organs, and the large muscle groups of the body.

- Affects each section of the spine and all the other joints of the body.

- Massages the abdominal and pelvic organs, especially ovaries.

Precautions and Contraindications:

- Pregnant women are advised to only do simple balance poses, such as tree pose. Also, since a balance pose can actually be harder than it looks, if you have a heart condition or high blood pressure, be careful.

- Those with low back, knee, ankle, or hip pain should begin by lying on the floor.

Half Shoulder Stand/Elevation
Sanskrit name: Ardha Sarvangasana

In this pose, your tailbone and feet are turned up to the sky as the physical determination of the spine remains erect, surrendering the will of the ego. The neck, throat, and third eye are grounded, releasing control to unleash your inner wisdom and trust in the universe. How much are you willing to let go of?

Entry and Holding Posture

1. Begin lying on your back with the body lengthened.

2. Place your arms at your sides with your palms down, and let your shoulders fall away from your ears.

3. Engage your abdomen, pulling your navel into your spine, and lift your legs straight at a 90-degree angle.

4. Place your hands under the backs of your hips. Press your elbows into the earth and, using your hands to support your pelvis, roll the hips off the earth.

5. Position your hands under your pelvis so the base of the palm cups the lower back crest to support the weight of the body evenly while tractioning the spine.

6. Bend your knees toward your forehead, then push up, straightening the legs and flexing the feet.

7. Align your forearms parallel to each other and distribute the weight evenly across both hands. If there is too much pressure on the arms, allow the legs to angle toward the head.

8. Press your shoulders away from each other to open your heart and take pressure away from your neck.

9. Release the pose by tucking the knees toward the forehead and rolling down the spine, one vertebra at a time.

Hold up to 15–30 seconds, or about five big breaths through the nostrils only.

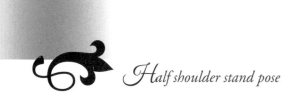

Half shoulder stand pose

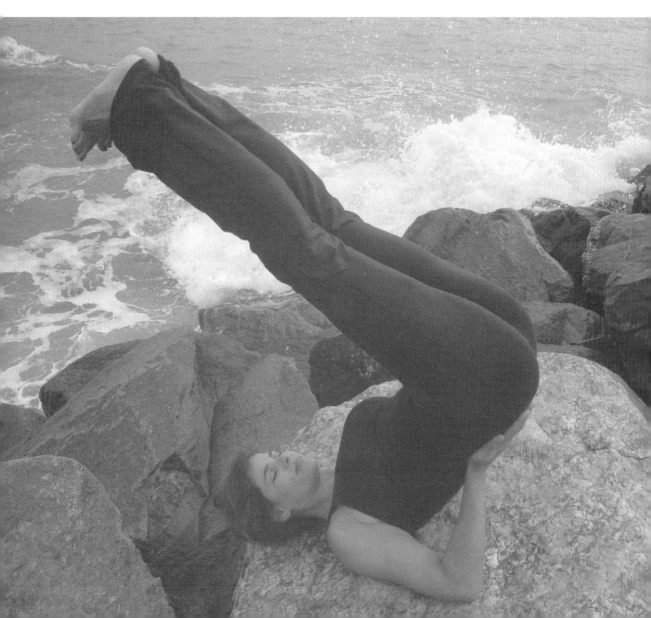

Benefits and Systems Being Treated, Challenged, and Healed:

- Strengthens the abdomen, hips, and legs, and provides pelvic stability.

- Regulates blood pressure.

- Brings blood to the face and brain for increased vitality.

- Massages thyroid and thymus.

- Strengthens lymphatic and circulatory systems.

- Reverses the position of all the internal organ, regulating their functions.

Precautions and Contraindications:

- Those with neck, shoulder, or wrist pain, high blood pressure, heart disease, stroke, hiatal hernia.

Modifications

- Use the wall for support, with one leg bent, taking strain off wrists and shoulders.

- Use blanket under shoulders to maintain the natural curve of the neck.

$\mathcal{P}$*low pose*

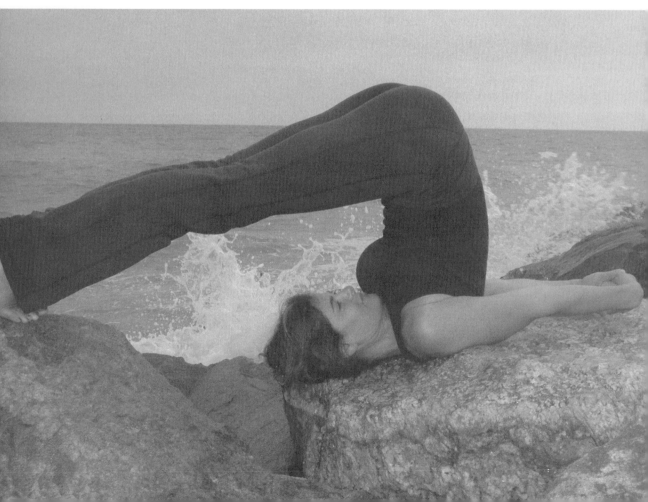

Plow / Growth

SANSKRIT NAME: HALASANA

The plow breaks and turns over the hard earth to fertilize and nourish new growth. A strong body and mind are needed to plow through a hard heart and to work out unhealthy thoughts. This creates more space to grow. Are you willing to do the work?

Entry and Holding Posture

1. Begin lying on your back with your body fully lengthened.

2. Place your arms at your sides with your palms down, and relax the shoulders away from the ears.

3. Engage your abdomen, pulling your navel into your spine, and lift your legs straight at a 90-degree angle.

4. Place your hands under the backs of your hips. Press your elbows into the earth and, using your hands to support the pelvis, roll the hips off the earth.

5. Position your hands under the pelvis so that the base of the palms cup the lower back crest to support the weight of the body evenly while tractioning the spine.

6. Bend your knees toward your forehead, then push up, straightening the legs and flexing the feet.

7. Align your forearms parallel to each other and distribute the weight evenly across both hands. If there is too much pressure on the arms, allow your legs to angle toward your head.

8. Press your shoulders away from each other to open your heart and take pressure off the neck.

9. Bring your legs over you, touching the floor with your feet. Separate your feet to take pressure off the neck and spine, then walk your feet together for a deep stretch and expression of posture.

10. Release the pose by tucking your knees toward the forehead and rolling down the spine, one vertebra at a time.

Hold up to 15–30 seconds, or about five big breaths through the nostrils only.

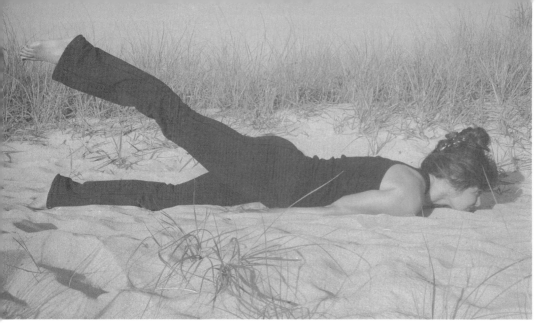

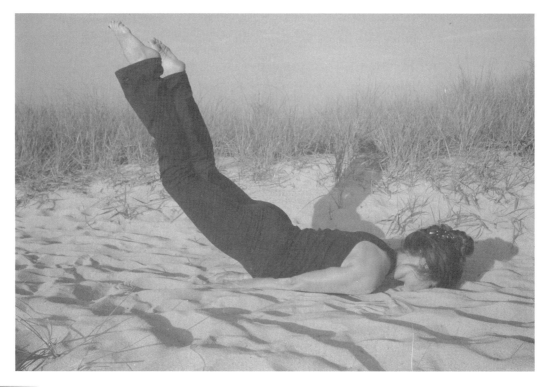

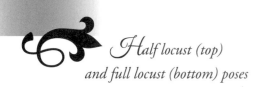 *Half locust (top) and full locust (bottom) poses*

Benefits and Systems Being Treated, Challenged, and Healed:

- Massages the spinal cord.

- Reverses the positions of all the internal organs, regulating their functions.

- Provides a deep massage for the kidneys, adrenal glands, diaphragm, and all the abdominal organs.

- Calms the brain.

- Stimulates the abdominal organs and the thyroid gland.

- Stretches the shoulders and spine.

- Helps relieve the symptoms of menopause.

- Reduces stress and fatigue.

- Therapeutic for backache, headache, infertility, insomnia, and sinusitis.

- Relaxes the fight-or-flight response and reprograms the nervous system.

Precautions and Contraindications:

- Weak back or neck muscles.

Half Locust/Concentration
Sanskrit name: Salambhasana

Are you weighed down by held-in emotions? Do you resist feeling your emotions for fear of being overwhelmed by their presence? How can you fly if you are weighed down by fear and doubt? How can you concentrate and remain focused if the restricted chatter of the mind outweighs the expansiveness and freedom of the heart? The mind will not allow what the heart wants to feel. Can you concentrate on releasing your fears?

Entry and Holding Posture

1. Lie flat on your stomach with chin to the floor, arms alongside the body, palms facing downward.

2. Slide your hands under your thighs with the palms and forearms pressed into the floor. If too hard, leave your arms and hands at the side of your thighs.

3. Press your pelvis and engage your arms by pressing them into the floor.

4. Inhale slowly, raise the right leg off the floor, and lengthen through your toes while pressing your hips down into the floor.

5. Chin still in contact with the floor, release leg slowly, using resistance bringing the leg to the floor.

6. Repeat with left leg.

7. Remove your hands from under your thighs and place the arms alongside your body.

8. Turn your head to the side and rest.

Hold up to 15–30 seconds each side, or about five big breaths through the nostrils only.

Full Locust Variation

1. Mouth to the floor.

2. Repeat steps as above.

3. Pressing your palms and forearms into the floor to give you strength, lift both legs up.

4. While inhaling, using the back muscles, lift both the legs together slowly, raising the legs as high as possible.

5. Lengthen through the legs and toes, squeezing the buttocks for strength, and lift.

Hold up to 15–30 seconds, or about five big breaths through the nostrils only.

Benefits and Systems Being Treated, Challenged, and Healed:

- Stimulates and tones abdominal muscles.

- Helps relieve stress.

- Tones thighs, buttocks, spine, and backs of arms and legs.

- Improves posture.

- Relieves constipation, indigestion, and flatulence.

- Relieves lower back pain.

- Strengthens the lungs.
- Stretches, strengthens, and creates flexibility in the shoulders, chest, belly, and thighs.

Precautions and Contraindications:
- Chronic injury to the back or weak back muscles
- Neck injury
- Serious back injury
- Headache

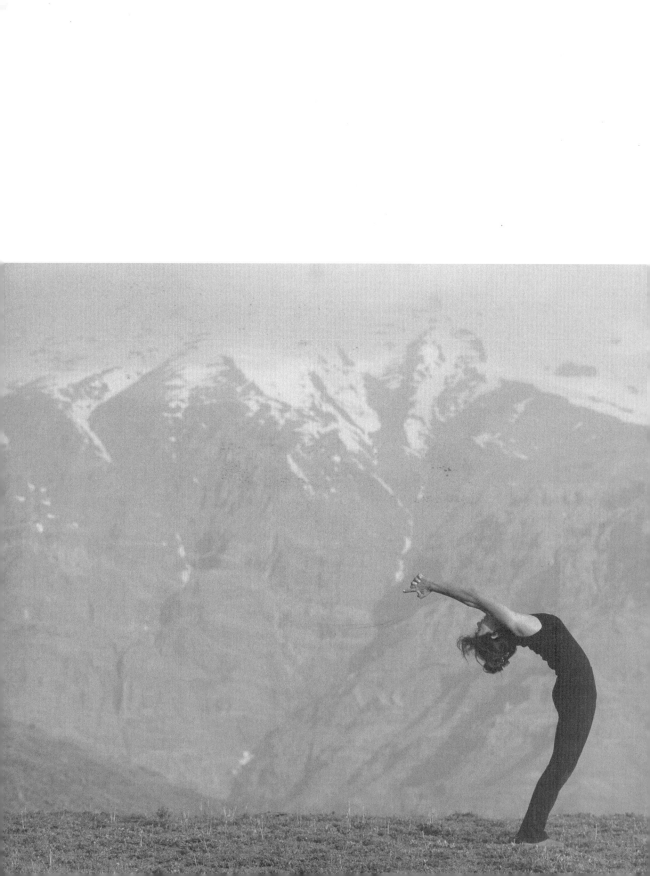

Chapter 4

THE EMOTIONAL BODY

Stress—a major cause of not allowing yourself to feel your emotions— has become the most potent poison in the world. Because we are constantly occupied with worrying about the future or regretting the past, we have become worriers instead of warriors. Stress takes up so much of our attention that we are losing all self-awareness—and therefore the ability to heal ourselves.

Stress kicks off a downward spiral: you blame your job, your kids, your relationship, your financial situation, and on and on for whatever is triggering your stress and thereby assume the role of the victim. Approaching life as a victim hinders you from taking action. Through this neglect, you become a participant in your own dis-ease. When you are constantly focused on your stressors, you are spending too much time in your mental body and neglecting your physical, emotional, and spiritual bodies. You become irritable, angry, judgmental, and irrational. Your energy no longer radiates outward, it sucks up energy from the people around you in order to survive. You react instead of act. You make choices to save time instead of to save your health. Does any of this sound familiar? Most of us are stress addicts and don't even know it.

Our culture may be one of the smartest and richest on the planet, but we keep running away from our responsibility to heal ourselves. We are so caught up with always producing that we are not realizing the casualties in our own lives. The average American's

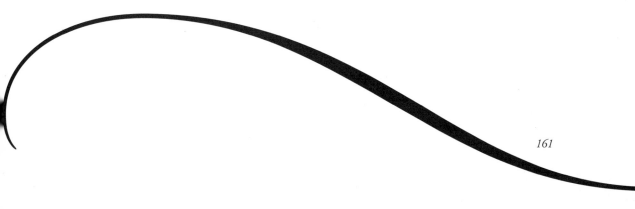

lifestyle is stressful to the point of being insane. We have become so distracted by daily stresses that we can no longer see and feel what is going on with each other and our environment. These dysfunctions have poisoned our minds, bodies, spirits, and souls and are a reflection of our inability to feel our emotions. We have become so concerned about how we look that we no longer know how we feel.

The belief "If I am thin and look good, everything is OK" is another form of daily stress. Thanks to the wonders of photo editing software, every photo of women we see in magazines has been retouched to the point where we no longer have a grasp of what is real and what is fake. The message we receive is, if you are beautiful, life is easier and you are worth more. There is nothing wrong with looking good, but not when it comes at the cost of feeling bad.

The irony is that trying to be perfect creates a lot of stress and actually causes us to age faster and deplete our life force. When we are stressed, we breathe shallowly, causing our energy levels to drop. We stop feeding the body the oxygen it needs to stay healthy, strong, and radiant. The body craves sugar and other stimulants because it is desperately seeking energy. As a result, our insulin levels rise and cue the body to store more fat. Other common results of stress are backaches, shortness of breath, irritability, hormonal imbalances, migraine headaches, unnecessary tension and anxiety, arthritis, wrinkles, insomnia, and fatigue. In this state, we also do not digest food properly, and our insides become a toxic waste dump. We lose our glow, our radiance, and become less sensitive to feeling our own energies and those around us. Stress also takes a toll on the nervous system, which then affects the ability of the immune system to work effectively. It's a downward spiral we must take steps to stop, or it will stop us.

This internal stress affects the largest organ: the skin. Our skin is the first organ to suffer from stress. We lose our glow and become desensitized as we start building emotional armor—a thick skin, as they say. This armor is an illusion of the mind that helps us feel less vulnerable. Yet if you want to stand in your true authentic self, you have to be willing to let go of the past and the future, and stand naked in the present moment.

When we take steps to eradicate stress and establish balance in all four of our bodies, we create natural beauty, health, and radiance inside and out. When we remove toxins and stress from our lives, we free our energy to rid us of anything that does not serve us. We also create an internal awareness to stop, look, listen, and feel. In this process, we find that sacred place inside us where everything is still, questions are asked, and answers are found—the place of self-love.

Taking time to reflect is a necessary daily practice to get rid of stress. It is just like brushing your teeth to get rid of plaque before it creates damage and disease. Creating time for reflection and stillness nourishes all four bodies: it releases toxins from the physical body, helps the mental body learn how to focus, creates an outlet for worries and pent-up feelings that create stress in our emotional body, and provides the quietness we need to hear the wisdom of all four bodies. We learn how powerful it is to surrender—to let go of old habits, patterns, beliefs, resentments, and worries to make room and allow the positive to come in. And as we surrender, all four of our bodies integrate, and we become whole once again. From this wholeness, we become balanced. And only when we are balanced can we reach our full potential.

Part of being human—and a woman in particular—is expressing your emotions. Denying your emotions denies your existence as a woman and your ability to evolve. It handicaps your emotional intelligence. It is no wonder that breast cancer and heart disease are climbing the charts as leading killers of women. We have denied our femininity, our emotions, our intuition, and our connection to each other and to Mother Earth.

In my retreats, one of the biggest awakenings is when the women in attendance learn how to be women again—how to express, not suppress; how to tap into their sensuality and sexuality from a pure place; how to be childlike and spontaneous again. Before the retreat, the women have become so rigid, they no longer flow like the water, dance like wildfire, let their hair down to be blown by the wind, or get dirty lying on the earth. Some women will not take their shoes off or will only sit on the ground if they are sitting on a blanket, not on the Mother herself.

When all of our senses are awakened, we feel the pleasure of being alive, sensual, powerful, and sexy—all aspects of a woman in tune with her femininity. I ask my boot camp attendees, what is your definition of sensuality and sexuality? And what does being feminine mean to you? Most have a hard time answering this question in a clear, precise manner. Our culture has distorted femininity, and we as women have distorted ourselves too. But if I asked what are your child's or partner's strengths, that would be a much easier question since it is not about them.

When you are in tune with your emotions, desires, and pleasures, you have the freedom to flow. When you have the freedom to flow, you have flexibility in all four bodies. When you have this flexibility, you have full range of motion to attract the abundance of love, health, wealth, and success. But in order to create this flexibility, you must first let go of what no longer serves you, including old emotional patterns, to allow the new to come in. Otherwise, you will just keep creating the same old story with new actors and actresses. To be an enlightened being, you must build the muscles of the emotional body, starting with emotional intelligence.

As you embark on this undertaking, use the following twelve rules as your trail markers along the way:

1. I will not deny my femininity. An emotionally immature woman is one who tries to act like a man and denies her own femininity and feminine essence to succeed, survive, or please others.

2. I will learn how to choose what I will or will not allow in my space and be responsible for it.

3. I will not deny my emotions because others are not in tune with theirs.

4. I am not being weak or a pushover for acting from my feminine core.

5. I will never mistake my kindness for weakness.

6. I will stop being a victim. Energy from the past is a drain on the present.

7. I will express, not suppress. Emotions are a part of existence. It takes more energy to hold emotions than to release them.

8. I will stop building other people's dreams and kingdoms. Instead, I will invest in myself.

9. I believe that my time, energy, and money are are worthy and equal to that of others.

10. Chaos and drama drain me energetically, emotionally, and financially.

11. How others perceive and filter what I do or say is not my responsibility as long as I speak with spiritual integrity.

12. Pleasure is not about what I have but how I feel.

I wish I had known these guidelines when I was growing up. It took years of self-reflection to come up with these guidelines for myself. I could have saved myself a lot of pain, money, and energy. Growing up, there were so many mixed messages all around me that I felt torn in several pieces. With all this stress and pressure, my body image started changing. I thought I wasn't good enough or attractive enough. I looked to women's magazines for guidance. I would compare myself to the girls in the magazines. I doubted myself as a girl and as a human being. Food became my new friend. I became obsessed with an unhealthy image of women and ended up gaining a lot of weight. I ate to swallow my emotions, then starved myself by suffering with bulimia and anorexia. I swallowed my pain with food and then was upset with myself for doing so.

Everyone would tell me, "You have such a pretty face—if only you could lose weight." My boyfriend told me I acted like a guy and I needed to be more feminine. Starting freshman year, I played varsity softball, basketball, and volleyball. There was always a goal and a deadline attached to whatever I did. The more pressure I felt, the more my eating disorders got worse. I was losing my hair, my fingers turned yellow from the stomach acid when I threw up, and I had massive migraine headaches. No one knew about my problem or even much about these diseases at that time.

I prayed for a way out and fantasized about being free, but I couldn't take care of myself or even sleep well because I was constantly on an adrenaline high. I was the sickest healthiest person I knew. The eating disorders were hard to hide, which I then masked with obsessive exercise and dieting, counting every calorie, going to the gym twice a day, and beating my body to a pulp—after all, no pain, no gain—all to maintain a so-called beautiful body, which I had on the outside, yet my insides were a mess. I had insomnia, addictive behaviors, ADD, and a couple more acronyms that our medical system made up. And the sad part of it all was that I was never taught how to work with my emotions.

I lost lots of weight and began modeling, which only fed my distorted body image even more. The women models I met looked nothing like their photos; the pressure to remain thin was unbearable and torturous. It was then, thank God, I realized the beauty industry was all an illusion, and I had to ask myself whether how I was hurting myself was worth the price. Ever wonder why our culture has the highest rate of depression, addiction, and abuse, while indigenous cultures that have not been tainted by our religious and cultural beliefs do not have these illnesses? They may be poor financially, but they are rich in heart, spirit, and soul.

Here are some questions you need to ask yourself: How many hours do you spend replenishing yourself each day? Each week? Think of how much energy you put out; are you taking in an equal amount? Would you not think the scale is tipped and at some point it will take its toll?

Although this chapter is about emotions, it also vitally important that we address money. You must understand that when you are emotionally drained, you are financially drained. Ever notice this in your life? When you are emotionally drained, you cannot manifest your basic needs and desires to survive and be happy. You put yourself in a constant state of stress and anxiety, creating a scarcity mentality, which puts you in an emotional tailspin. When you realize your energy equals time and time equals money, you can make healthier choices and investments in yourself, creating an energetic account of self-worth consistently flowing and filled with vitality and the abundance of love, health, wealth, success, and beauty, inside and out. Women as a whole are burnt out because we do not understand the value of our gifts, which puts us in a constant state of overdraft and of being overextended emotionally and physically.

You can look at relationships in this way, too. How many times have you not listened to your intuition? You knew you should not have gotten into a relationship or a situation, yet you did it anyway, thinking you could help. You invested all your time, your emotions, and your entire self wholeheartedly, yet it ended up being a setback because you did not listen to your emotional intelligence and your intuition, the major gifts of a balanced and powerful goddess. How many years and how much money did you invest, and was it worth it in the end? All because you did not trust your inner wisdom. Ladies, wake up. What we have to share is not tangible. It's our energy, our love, our time; you can't put a price tag on it. You have to ask, how much am I worth? If time equals money, then your energy equals time *and* money.

We must learn how to use our energy, not be used by it. In order to learn this valuable lesson, we must be able to understand this simple equation. Where does our energy begin and where does it end? What will you allow or not allow into your space, not only physically but energetically? In order to learn these tools, we must know how to set healthy boundaries, not create walls.

I hear many women blaming their partner for their failed relationship, but this is a cop-out. It's just as much about you as it is about the other person. After all, you chose them; they are only a reflection of you. When you realize this truth, you can heal and grow much faster than if you stay stuck in your anger and victimhood. It is all about you and why you do the things you do. Ask yourself what you are doing, why you are doing it, and how it is affecting you. When you can answer these basic questions, you are on your way to healing. You start to ask yourself, why did I pick this in my life? How did I create this as my reality? How do I heal it? How do I remain in my integrity for myself? Why did I not stand in my truth? How did I lose myself?

When you can take responsibility and answer these questions, you heal faster and are grateful for the gifts that person taught you, no matter how painful they were. First you will be angry, then you will grieve, and then, if you are able to surrender, you will forgive. If you don't get to forgiveness, you must remember that the person who hurt you will still have control over your life, because you will still give your thoughts, emotions, and time to this situation. You do not have this kind of free time, nor do you want to allow someone else to control your life. If you continue to concentrate on this situation—this person, place, or thing you are not healing—you are giving your energy and time to a useless cause.

When you stop, look, listen, and feel the pain instead of running from it, you no longer feed it. The energy will dissipate since you are not feeding it, and you can climb the emotional intelligence scale to love—the emotion with the highest frequency. What frequency do you choose to live in—anger and victimhood, or freedom and love? It is always a choice.

There is no knight in shining armor. In our new version, the princess saves herself. Do not get caught in the illusion of love; instead, choose the reality of love.

Spiritual Body
Honor Your True Nature
Where, when, and how did you first disconnect from the source of God's love? What part of you does not feel worthy of love?

Mental Body
Learn the Discipline of Silence and Stillness
What are the belief systems that either take you closer or further away from the source of this love?

Emotional Body
Give Yourself Permission to Feel
What are the ways you have punished or hurt yourself so that you do not feel worthy of love?

Physical Body
Build a Foundation of Strength and Stamina
Why do you keep creating the same story that does not feed you this love or connect you to the source of this love?

Loving yourself first is the healthiest gift you can give to someone—a centered, whole, healthy being who is able to protect, provide, and love herself without need or want, manipulation, or sacrifice—the very things we have been taught that love is. It is time to put your female spirit into action to create what you desire, require, and deserve. And in order to do this, you must first create boundaries, not walls, meaning you must develop the ability to sense energy and set limitations on outside influences that take you further away from your authentic, divine self. And if that means standing alone, then that is exactly what you need to do for yourself, your sanity, your health, and your children. Your first and foremost lover and friend is Mother Earth and Spirit. Everything else is a reflection of this relationship.

Goddess of the Emotional Body:
DURGA

Descriptors
FOR THIS GODDESS

Also known as Devi to the Indians and Diva to the Italians—from the Latin word *diva*, meaning "goddess," the feminine version of *divus*, meaning "god."

Strong, graceful, centered, balanced, courageous, self-reliant

Message from This Goddess [18]

When threatened by demons, I fiercely protect myself with all that I have from deep within. I call forth all that I need. I am inaccessible, for I place myself beyond the reach of all that would destroy me and all that try to wound me. I am the unapproachable, for nothing can get at me that I do not willingly let in. I dance my dance of oneness only with what supports me, nurtures me, and loves me. For all that does not, I say: approach at your own risk.

---

18 Used with permission from Amy Sophia Marashinsky's *The Goddess Oracle* (U.S. Games Systems, 2006).

How This Goddess Works in Your Life

Were you taught to be nice? When you expressed your emotions or feelings of frustration or anger, were you told you were not being a nice girl? Were you taught to put others before you, to not hit or defend yourself, to take up less space because you were a girl? Do you feel pulled consistently off your center by giving too much of yourself?

I remember one night in boot camp, one of the women introduced me and the other goddesses to her husband. He had us all in stitches talking about men as they get older, how they finally surrender their egos and realize how powerful their women are. He told us, "I do not understand; as little boys and men, we are always following you and wanting to be in your space. Where did you lose that power over us?" We had that power at one time: not power *over* but the power of self-love. Where did we become selfless and "lesser than"? We have lost the ability to defend ourselves verbally because we were taught to be nice girls, to make the world a nicer place, to keep our anger contained. As the saying goes, if you have nothing nice to say, do not say it all. Women in past generations were taught the belief system of not being smarter or stronger than men because it would bruise their egos and they would never find a husband this way. And even today, some women make more money than their partner does, which can create a problem in the relationship. But why should a woman feel guilty or pay a price for being her best and powerful self?

If you do not know your basic needs, how do you expect others to? You must ask yourself what your boundaries are—what are the rules and guidelines for yourself and others to abide by? What does your center feel like? How in Goddess's name are you going to know what power feels like if you do not know how to claim your own space? What threw you off your center and why? Where do you stand, and do you know how to take a stand? Where do you start and others begin?

If you lose your sense of self, you also lose the ability to protect and provide for yourself. You become energetic food for others and fall prey to predators. You must know how to use your energy, not be used by it. This is a sign of codependent behavior. You cannot be open in your heart and not be present and grounded in your body.

Most girls are taught to have an open heart and be kind, compassionate, and nice. This learned behavior comes at their own expense, because they then have no ability to set boundaries and filter out predators. They are taught that their bodies are for others' pleasure and that their worth is derived from what they look like. If you do not believe me, take a look at almost every show on TV. Sex sells, meaning the exploitation of women sells. Our feminine essence is a commodity to those who want to abuse it. The press, the media, the fashion and beauty industries, even our peers constantly remind us that our beauty is our foremost asset. You do not hear boys being told "You are so handsome" by someone they just met. This emphasis on looks is a cultural hazard.

You did not come here to sleep but to be awake. You did not come here to live in pain but to experience pleasure. You did not come here to be still but to dance. You did not come here to take up space but to claim it.

What Is the Emotional Body?
GIVE YOURSELF PERMISSION TO FEEL

The emotional body, also known as the pranic body in the yoga tradition, is ruled by the water element. Water is the blood of Mother Earth. Like the spiritual body and the mental body, the emotional body is intangible and nondimensional. It holds the energetic blueprint of all of our experiences, otherwise known as our baggage. It digests, assimilates, and integrates internal and external information and brings forth awareness. This awareness stimulates the nervous system's fight-or-flight response and all five senses, which then triggers sensations, feelings, and vibrations. These stimuli lead to an emotional response that is stored not only in the memory of our minds but also in our DNA, creating cellular memory.

The emotional body is the hardest body to get in shape and keep in shape since it holds the archives of all of our experiences. It is intertwined with the seven chakras, the wheels of energy located along the spine that connect the energetic, intangible bodies—the spiritual, mental, and emotional bodies—to the physical body.

These chakras are receptors that take in and release energy from the environment and universe. They are like pumps that regulate the flow of energy through our emotional body and affect how we perceive something, how we feel, and how we think. The seven chakras are the seven different colors of the rainbow, each with its own vibration of sound, smell, sensation, and taste. They are also each connected to an organ, gland, body part, and emotion. The power of the chakras cannot be overstated: they create our reality by affecting how we perceive what is going on within and around us.

Since the emotional body stores memories, it creates new ones based on what it has experienced already. This is why it is very hard to break a bad habit or change your thinking. You have to confront your issues stored in your tissues, otherwise you will continually repeat them, attracting new actors and actresses to play out the same emotional scene over and over again. That scene is like watching a TV show, whether it be a drama, action series, dysfunctional reality show, or a heart-wrenching love story; we have to be able to step back and observe our self in the scene, and what part we play and how we are creating our reality in the moment. When we can recognize and take responsibility for the part we play, we can change the station and create a new story with a happier and functional ending. This strength is emotional intelligence, which keeps the emotional body healthy, therefore giving us the ability to erase cellular memory. Because you are no longer accepting this as your reality or truth, you are no longer playing victim or perpetrator, therefore no longer feeding the pain and dysfunction.

In order to heal, you must feel. You must validate your emotions and understand that their intelligence is as valid as any other intelligence. To be book smart, you must study; to be emotionally intelligent, you must feel, validate, and deal with your emotions.

Examples of How the Emotional Body Works

You may try and will your way through something—giving up smoking, for example, or changing your diet—but resistance is stored in the emotional body: your energy field, your senses, and your cells. You may be successful for thirty days, or even six months, but those same old bad habits will creep back in, because the information that's stored in your emotional body will always lead you to repeat your old behavior whenever you experience a stressful situation. If you are trying to quit smoking and you lose your job, all your old triggers come back. The sound of a lighter, the flare of a just-lit cigarette, the smell of the smoke, the taste of an alcoholic beverage that always accompanied your cigarette. All of your senses create a response in your mind and body, causing you to lose control and then feel ashamed for failing.

You did not fail, you just have to use your emotional intelligence. You have to ask yourself, why did I ever pick up that cigarette in the first place? Did you want to look cool or calm your nerves or boost your self-esteem? Whatever the reason, every time that same emotion comes creeping back into your life, you will respond to it the same way. And the more often you respond in the same way, the more the tissues of your body will hold the memory. You have to ask yourself why. The cigarette is a crutch. It represents the part of you that has lost itself and disconnected from the source of love, all because you did not want to deal with your emotions at the time.

The body is 80 percent water, the strongest element. It can wear down steel, rock, and mountains, as evidenced by the Grand Canyon, the mountains of Patagonia, the glaciers of Antarctica, the waterfalls of Hawaii, and every ocean, sea, lake, and river. Even our own life force, our blood, is made up of water. Water also conducts energy, which creates electricity.

Women retain more water in their bodies than men because we are more intuitive. It is a gift. This water within us ignites our intuitive abilities, giving us the ability to sense and feel energy on another level. It allows us to be more in tune with the seen and unseen worlds. It is when we do not use this natural psychic ability that we create our own pain. Our energy becomes stagnant, which is painful and emotionally paralyzing.

Most women cannot lose weight or get off their antidepressants because they are not allowing their emotions and their energy to flow. They are carrying emotional baggage and years of suppressed emotions. Only when they finally release it does their energy flow naturally.

I receive phone calls and emails all the time from women who say they lost thirty pounds without even thinking about it. I always laugh because I know they lost the baggage they had been carrying for years. They validated their emotions, faced their fears, and claimed their feminine essence, reigniting the fire and electricity within. They reclaimed the most powerful part of themselves: being in tune with their emotions and listening to their intuition.

When you run from your emotions and turn off your intuition, you separate yourself from your body and become a slave to your mind. Only when you are in your body can you experience pleasure—whether it's from food, nature, other people, or the union with a loved one. Stuffing your emotions becomes heavy on an energetic level, which then affects the physical body. The metabolism slows down, you store more body fat, and it takes an enormous amount of energy just to move. You may notice that it takes three lattes just to get going every day. Just as water needs to flow, so do our emotions and our energy. You start to get fed up with yourself, until finally the pain of staying where you are becomes worse than feeling what your emotional body has to tell you.

Muscles of the Emotional Body

Sensation

Sensation provides awareness of energy, whether it's through sound, touch, taste, smell, or sight. Sensations (hot, cold, numb, tingling, bright, uncomfortable) are signals of what is going on within the body. These sensations tell us how energy is moving or not moving in the body. The skin is most sensitive to sensation and is the thermostat of the body, the temperature-control system, and also the largest organ of the body.

Feelings

Feelings bring forth internal awareness. A feeling is not a reaction—rather, emotions are the responses we have to feelings. A feeling can be an intuitive understanding, a physical impression on the skin such as touch, a mental recognition of understanding, or an intuitive gut feeling.

Vibration

Vibration is the speed and density at which energy moves—whether it is fast, slow, heavy, or light. Vibration is the result of the movement of energy that creates a sensation and feeling.

You may have said about someone, "She is giving off a bad vibe." You can sense and feel others' energy by the tone of their voice, facial expressions, body language, and the words that come out of their mouth. All give off a vibration that gives you information to determine what course of action you are going to take—whether you will move into or move away from it.

Frequency

Frequency is a measurable rate of a motion, whether it be sound, electricity, or electromagnetic energy. Just as there are frequencies of sound, light, and color, there are frequencies of emotions. Everyone can tell the difference between an angry person and a joyful person by their facial expressions, body language, and the energy they project. You can feel the frequency of anger being lower than joy. Which one do you want to be around, and which one do you choose to live by? An atom emits a glow of light. The radiant field, or the body of light, demonstrates the health of a cell, which resonates a frequency. Everything alive has a frequency that we can measure through our senses of touch, sight, sound, taste, and smell. It only makes sense, then, that the food we eat, the environment we live in, and the people we surround ourselves with can either feed and speed up our frequency or slow us down. (We will discuss this more in the physical body chapter.)

Conscious living supports the systems of the body to function properly and to our maximum potential, which is the zero point. We must learn that our physical body operates like electricity, which feeds our electromagnetic field and in return runs through every cell of our organs, glands, and systems like electricity giving off a vibration, which creates a frequency.

Emotions

Emotions are the essence of being human. They separate us from the animal, plant, and mineral kingdoms. The word *emotion* means "energy in motion" in Latin. It is also related to the word *motivation*, which means "to act."

Emotions give off internal and external responses that can affect our well-being. Internally, our emotions stem from the heart and mind releasing adrenaline, endorphins, and other natural hormones that can create harmony or chaos in all the major systems in our body, such as circulatory, respiratory, lymphatic, skeletal, endocrine, muscular, and digestive.

Externally, our emotions stem also from the mind and heart, releasing harmony and peace or stress and angst. Both can be visually seen and energetically felt by our posture, facial expressions, glow in the eyes, and overall appearance and presence, which all reflect a mindset of healthy self-esteem and self-worth or victimhood and martyrdom.

Emotional Intelligence

Emotional intelligence is our ability and willingness to learn, understand, and recognize emotions, not only as responses to feelings but as energy that can be used to challenge, treat, and heal the human species. As I discussed in the mental body, the right side of the brain's functions are feminine aspects—creativity, intuition, and receptivity. It also holds emotional memories and recognizes patterns. In order to heal, we must go deeper into our holistic and intuitive self to tap into our emotional intelligence.

FIRST STEP: Because emotions are energy, you first have to be able to sense it, feel it, and acknowledge it before you can access it.

SECOND STEP: Recognize that love is not just an emotion but also a powerful force that has action behind it. There is no separation between good and evil, love and hate; it all comes from the same source. Your perception creates an emotional response.

PERCEIVE THIS: If everything is made from the same source, the love of God, and we are God, then how can there be separation? Separation comes when the mind will not allow what the heart wants to feel. If all is made from this love, then all can be healed from this love.

Even in the darkest emotions there is light and awareness. What you do with this awareness is the result of a choice between faith or fear. Your emotional intelligence makes this choice. Even the blackest feathers of a crow or raven still reflect light. Even the abyss of our mind reflects light, where all creation is born.

How you perceive things dictates what you believe. This belief will have a sensation, a feeling, and a frequency that will give off a vibration and ultimately a reaction, leading to an emotional response. How, when, and where you release this emotional response is emotional intelligence.

Each emotion has its own frequency. When you can recognize where emotions fall on the spectrum of frequencies, you build your emotional intelligence. But first you must understand the basics of the emotion with the highest frequency: love. This emotion aims for improvement, not perfection. The only thing that is perfect is Spirit, and Spirit created us all different so that we can express all the innumerable aspects of love.

THE SCALE OF EMOTIONS

When you can practice validating, feeling, and dealing with your emotions, you can heal. Again, you must feel to heal. Your emotions are like notes played by musical instruments, from the deep rumblings of the drum to the soft sound of the chimes. Each emotion carries a frequency that can be pleasant or annoying, all depending on where you are at in your life. Learning to work with the scale of emotions can help you determine how to work with your own symphony of emotions.

Emotion—Feeling—Action—Reaction

Unconditional love—unlimited devotion—nonjudgment for self and others—judgmental of self and others

Joy—sense of well-being—expression of healthy and vital spirit—lack of vitality and excitement for life

Peace—calmness, freedom from distraction—no more drama or chaos—overstimulated and reactive

Contentment—ease and satisfaction—finding and living from your gift of God, your purpose—lack of motivation

Boredom—searching for purpose—understanding how you can be of service to Spirit; when you are of service to Spirit, you are of service to self—lifeless

Self-love—sense of self and devotion to self-worth—living from your true authentic self—codependent, living through others, lack of self; victim (powerless), martyr (poor me), perpetrator (controlling)

Forgiveness—letting go—creating space within for new opportunites and abundance—hatred, stagnant, stuck, lack of empathy for self and others

Grief—sorrow, distress—validating feelings of loss to release, purify, and detox mind, body, and spirit—lack of feeling leading to depression

Rage, anger—sadness, madness, injustice, displeasure—expression of deep hurt and pain—suppressed emotions, self-abusive

Apathy—lack of interest in life—numb to feelings, emotions, and sensations—paralyzed by fear

I came up with this scale for myself to help me reach the peak of my true potential. It helped keep my mind focused and my heart open to rate my experiences and decide where I wanted to live on the scale. Did I want to continually be a victim of my emotions? I needed to learn how to harness them and use them to my best ability. I needed to defeat my inner demons—my fears—and in doing so, I needed a plan, and this scale is what worked for me. It still does for me and for many of my clients.

When you can ride the wave of emotions, you can determine whether they are a tsunami or a canoe trip down a calm river. Do you want to be known as a Drama Queen or an empowered Goddess Warrior? When you know how emotions work, you can create change.

Here are some guidelines to be mindful of when dealing with your emotions:

- Feelings are not facts—they can change.

- Feelings are not what people relapse over; the response and reactions are.

- Addiction is a disease caused by not being able to handle your feelings.

- You won't die from crying, but you might die from stress or addiction.

- Love is action; fear is reaction.

- Love expands; fear contracts.

- Love takes action; fear paralyzes.

- Situations may be different but feelings are the same.

- Codependence is the result of identifying someone else's needs and feelings
  as your own.

Climbing the scale of emotions can be quite empowering. You learn to observe your responses and ask yourself, *am I reacting or acting*? Are you acting like the twelve-year-old girl who fears speaking her truth and becomes angry and frustrated, or are you the forty-four-year-old woman who stands in her truth and feels her sense of self-worth? Feelings are timeless. It does not matter when one of your emotional triggers happens, it only matters how you act or react, because your triggers will continually repeat until you understand how to change it.

Women have many stresses and illnesses, yet most do not realize how numb they are. They are frustrated because they fear their emotions are too powerful to release. They have become such great actresses and chameleons that they have lost their sense of self. When I start the shifting process of getting to the abundance of love within them, they are scared of releasing, because they feel it will never end. They fear the rage and anger that is underneath their pain, because women are taught anger and rage are not nice. Because they feel safe in a supporting, nonjudgemental space, they are able to break free from the "nice girl syndrome" and allow their anger and rage to surface from the depths of their bellies and yonis (vagina and female reproductive system), where these deep emotions have settled from swallowing them for years. They soon realize that many women are going through the same emotions and that their pain is one and an injustice to their female essence. And when these deep-rooted emotions are validated, their desires are awakened, their hearts are open, and their bodies are free to experience pleasure.

I help them to understand that if you are numb and you express your anger, you have started climbing the scale of emotions and shifting to a higher frequency. After they feel that anger, then they can cry and release their sadness, moving further up the scale. As they climb the scale, they feel forgiveness for themselves and realize how brutally they have treated themselves and others. They then realize they will not tolerate any behavior that hurts them spiritually, mentally, emotionally, or physically. They find their worth and learn where their energy begins and ends. The fire of rage that once depleted and paralyzed them now feeds them the strength to move forward and create change. The way they allowed themselves to be treated shifts, and they feel the power of their own presence. They feel alive and wonder how they ever allowed themselves to live at such a low frequency. They understand how easy it is to follow this emotional workout and look forward to going deeper. There is no more paralyzing fear, because they know they can now defeat their fears.

They want to share this freedom with others. They know they are not here to take up space but to claim it. The goddess mantra is embedded in every cell of their being:

> *I am a twenty-first-century goddess.*
> *I am feminine*
> *I am sensual*
> *I am sexual*
> *I am powerful*
> *Don't ever mistake my kindness for weakness,*
> *And don't ever take me for granted.*

Remember, empowerment means pulling forth what is already within you. In order to find it, you must go inward and pull the best of yourself forward, even if it gets ugly at times. There is so much beauty, even in the worst of times.

The women then want to share their newfound wisdom, and this is how we as goddesses create change.

This is one of many stories of women who have come into alignment with Spirit with the 4 Body Fit concept of Boot Camp for Goddesses.

GODDESS STORY

I was drawn to Boot Camp for Goddesses by a description in a brochure, and it wrought changes in me I had not believed possible. I had suffered from fibromyalgia for more than eight years. At times I was so wholly debilitated that I could not lift my body to sit. I could walk only with a cane. Only forty-six, I felt more like sixty—I was unable to run with my children and had to ride in a wheelchair through the airports.

The brochure was ripe with descriptions of things I loved or thought I would; the breath was sucked out of me when I read the line, "for women of all fitness levels." I knew I had to be there. All fitness levels, all fitness levels—it became a mantra as I signed up and prepared to go; "all fitness levels" meant me! And it was true.

At the beginning of the week, I could do only minimal activities, pulling myself along the smallest part of the hiking trail with a walking stick and grasping at tree branches. By the end of week, I made the whole trail. Within a month, I returned to that same trail and, in 104-degree heat, traversed the entire thing, passing up my tennis-player friend who was huffing to keep up with me! How this happened is both a miracle and a simple reality.

My friends ask me, "That all happened in just one week? How is that possible?" It began on the first full day with simple yet intensive breathwork. Sierra instructed us to invite previous generations of women into the room. At first, I breathed into a body that was stuck and congested. The touch of my partner, the encouragement of Sierra, and my steady breathing finally brought me to tears. Tumbling in came realizations about me and my illness, as well as the various illnesses and limitations of my mother and her mother and the generations before her. I wept for us, for what we had been through and what we had done. Then came the shocking realization: we had done this to ourselves. We had all taken so much responsibility—often in arrogance, taking on what was not ours—that the only way to achieve the essential rest that our bodies and souls required was to create an illness. Only in this way were we temporarily excused from the duties of life. And we shored up on waves of sympathy.

Then someone new came into my consciousness, bringing a new message: my mentally disabled sister. She made it clear that her life was considerably happier when the family allowed her to move into her own home. Here was this girl-child, now a woman in her own right, communicating to me over space and time, saying as clear as day, "Do you see? I never wanted you to take care of me; that was the real burden to me. Now I'm free." Seeing her there, among my mother, my grandmothers, and myself, she was the only one who was healthy and wholly herself. The glorious contradiction of it, like a good joke, was suddenly funny—all that mistaken belief over the years—and I began to laugh. I laughed and laughed, loud and long and without restraint. Each time I began to stop, another image came to me: a face, a name, a dog, a memory of untying my grandmother's apron strings. I laughed at our silliness, thinking we knew what was what, even while we destroyed ourselves.

The more I saw, the more I laughed as the heavy years dropped away. My body eased with the release of it. My breath moved into my upper body for the first time, maybe ever. I felt warmth and glory, and a sense that I was healing back through the generations. I was humbled at the privilege of being the one there, lying on the floor, bathed in light.

My spiritual and emotional bodies had begun a new journey; now it was time for the mind and body to follow. The daily hikes and yoga poses helped, even if all I could do was lie on my side and stay present with my eyes. Transformation crept into me as I felt the flow of power moving through me. By the second night, I was too awake to go to bed. Clad only in a sarong, I was drawn out into the night alone. Sitting on a boulder in a grove of trees, I began to play a drum I had brought with me but had not played much before. It was unlike anything I had ever done before in my suburban existence: I began to drum and sing with the intent of beginning my magic, to seek healing from Mother Earth. Somehow, I felt she would honor the request. You must understand I have never done this before.

After another night and another day, I entered the womb of my first sweat lodge with a clear intention to face it all. Terrified but longing for release, I placed myself far from the exit. The door went down, and the universe opened up. After several minutes, my illness gripped my sides and I struggled to remain sitting. I heard a voice say, "You can sit up and burn it out of you, or you can lay your belly on me and let me heal you." I released a sigh, bared my belly, and lowered my body to the hard, cool earth. After a time of rest, I began to experience a vapor being drawn out of my belly, my solar plexus, down several feet into the ground. It went on and on, drawing out of me at a steady pace; after a time, I noticed that the lower part of my body felt good! The good-feeling part of my body grew as the gripped part shrank. I could feel health moving higher and higher, until the better part of me felt clear and renewed. At the end of that round, I left the lodge briefly to breathe the open air. When I glanced back at the door, suddenly all of me craved getting back in. I entered, reveling in the heat and the darkness for the fourth and final round, not knowing of the miracle about to occur. This time I sat upright and strong. For the first time in nearly ten years, the illness had left me; I was free.

The final day marked the next miracle: I made my first complete journey around the trail. I cannot begin to explain what that felt like, after so many years of limitation. At the end, I came upon a stone altar. I laid my walking stick upon it, said my thanks, and walked away. In the days that followed boot camp, I continued to heal. Final traces of restriction around my upper midsection, which I now knew how to breathe into, were released. Within another week, the restrictions were gone, and my physical and emotional endurance began building, actually moving forward from health into fitness. Yoga and walking were a joy. On longing for another interesting thing to do with this new body, I began training on the flying trapeze, now one of my greatest joys.

The gratitude I feel in every cell and muscle every day is greater for having experienced limitation for so long. Am I all that I can be? Not yet, and that is the best part. As I create new flexibility and strength in muscles long dormant, I find a continuing depth of spirit, solidity in relationships, and calm in the face of challenges, to stand on the ground and breathe the air. When weary or stressed, I now know to seek healing and connection from the earth and sky, to recognize the Goddess within, the Goddess beneath, and the Spirit that lives in all that surround me.—*Laura Faulkner, Ph.D.*

Boundaries

In order to tap into energy, you first have to be able to sense it, feel it, and acknowledge it. Boundaries are a verbal, physical, and energetic filter to keep unhealthy energies from invading your space. Verbally, you can express your discomfort; physically, you can move away; and energetically, you can repel it. When you learn what is comfortable for you and what is not, you can set boundaries according to what feels right for you.

Your energetic field is a three-foot sphere all around your physical body. Since your emotional body is an energetic body, it works very subtly. It can detect the vibrations and frequencies of energy in its space. If you have no sense of where your energy ends, your boundaries will be weak and you will become an energetic sponge, making you oversensitive to your environment because you do not know how to repel it. You have a hard time separating what you deserve and what you do not deserve, and you accept bad behavior from other people.

How you think is how you feel, how you feel is how you behave, and how you behave is what you will create. If you allow something into your space, then you must be responsible for the outcome.

If you don't have boundaries, you will create emotional armor to feed your story of being a victim. Emotional armor acts as a shield that stops you from receiving or giving energy because you feel vulnerable or not worthy. It is an illusion of protection that creates isolation over time, which leads to deep depression. The armor will shut down your energetic body and flow of life force. Diseases like arthritis, fibromyalgia, cysts, and fibroids are all held-in emotions that create resentment and victimization.

This armor cuts off your energy, intuition, and instincts, which in turns cuts off your five senses' ability to feel, see, hear, touch, or taste. Your energy becomes stagnant, thus becoming painful. You no longer put out energy or receive it; you just take up space instead of claiming it.

Karma

Karma means "deed" or "act" in Sanskrit. It refers to the universal principle of cause and effect, action and reaction, that governs all life. It is a spiritual law believed by Hindus and Buddhists. It is comparable to the admonishment inherent in the Ten Commandments: "Thou shalt be responsible for your own actions, and if thou do not follow the law of energy, there will be consequences."

The key to understanding karma lies in intelligent action and nonreactive response. As humans, we have free will to create our own destiny; karma is not fate. Because the emotional body stores the memories of our past hurts, pains, and joys, how we respond to the stimuli that surrounds us can create drama and chaos or calm and centeredness. To release heavy karmic issues such as addiction, abuse, and depression, you must be able to climb the scale of emotions and erase the reactive part of yourself, and take action to create the destiny that you desire, require, and deserve.

Many of us become lazy and give up our fate to the universe and then blame the universe when our prayers are not heard or don't happen quickly enough. We become victims because we keep score. Our attention span lessens, and we lose faith. But what we always seem to forget is that we must create the space to shift our karma. We must do the work of listening to our inner voice through meditation, asking for help through prayer, feeling all our emotions, and taking action. Karma does not mean we leave everything up to fate—that's a false perception the New Age movement has created. If you want Spirit to help, you must be willing to follow through and do the work.

When we are quiet enough to hear our intuition and inner voice, we can then hear God within us. And when we hear that internal voice, we receive direction, whether it is to move toward something or to be still and wait. Praying is then asking for help with the information you receive. Here's an example: On a walk in nature, I hear my inner voice tell me to leave my job. Then my fear sets in—what about money? I then pray for the strength and guidance to follow my intuition and place me where I need to be. I call in my guides, friends, and family for support and understanding. When we take the first step after hearing Spirit's call, the universe then takes us seriously and guides us to the next step. When you ask and receive your answer but do not follow through, then you are like the boy who cried wolf. Why would Spirit hear your prayer if you do not take the guidance seriously?

A Healthy Emotional Body

The emotional body is a filter, just as the spiritual body is. Its job is to know what it will or will not allow in its own personal space. It knows the balance of giving and receiving and does not judge others' emotions but knows what is healthy or unhealthy for it. A healthy emotional body knows overexerting the mind and body can cause adrenal fatigue, injuries, impaired performance, and emotional distress. A healthy emotional body knows how to balance effort and action with stillness and silence, action and reaction. It trusts innate wisdom, the instinct within us that knows the right choices and moves, the best timing, and helps us release detrimental stress by setting boundaries.

A healthy emotional body is sensitive to its environment yet not oversensitive to the chatter and noise around it. It expands and contracts with energy and breath. It is active, not reactive, when emotional buttons are pushed. It will not engage in verbal or energetic foreplay for the sake of winning. It realizes that energy equals time, and time equals money. It knows who is manipulating or pulling on your energy for their own needs. It can sense the energetic barnacles of lower frequencies trying to attach themselves to feed off your energy. It recognizes the energies of codependency and victim behavior. It will not fall victim to others because it knows where its energy ends and another begins. It has overall balance with its surroundings. It transforms energy instead of trying to control it. It is nonconfrontational; assertive, not aggressive. It knows that energy from the past is a drain on the present, and that it takes more energy to hold emotions than to release them.

Qualities
OF A HEALTHY EMOTIONAL BODY

Expands and contracts with energy and breath, energetic, self-reliant, clean, flexible, durable, nonjudgmental, transparent, active, in tune with emotions, expressive, willing to heal

The emotional body knows how to work with and create balance among the intellectual, native, and holistic energies within itself. It knows how to observe its environment with all its senses and knows what do with the information it receives. It radiates positive energy, coming from a higher frequency of emotions, yet it respects the purpose of lower ones.

A healthy emotional body takes responsibility for what circumstances it gets itself into and out of with truth and a sense of self, not blame and shame. It is willing to do the work and climb the scale of emotions to reach the peak of a true authentic self.

An Unhealthy Emotional Body

An unhealthy emotional body is oversensitive or insensitive, overstimulated or numb to others' feelings as well as its own. It either projects helplessness or tries to exert power over others for fear of not being loved and in control. It is too open and gives its energy away freely, or it shuts down or plays the victim. An unhealthy emotional body invades others' space because it does not know where it ends and another begins.

Because it does not know how to generate its own energy for itself or from its environment, it attaches itself to others for energy. An unhealthy emotional body is passive-aggressive. It suppresses emotions instead of expressing them, keeping the body in a constant state of fight-or-flight response, overloading the nervous system and adrenal glands, and creating a constant state of stress and fatigue.

Qualities OF AN UNHEALTHY EMOTIONAL BODY

Heaviness, pent-up emotions, addiction, abuse, codependency, reactivity, suppression, numbness, victimhood

When pain does not have an outlet, we become numb, weakening our senses, becoming prey to predators; this is the beginning of any addiction or depression that weakens the emotional body and immune system, in turn leaving us drained and ungrounded, leading to drama, chaos, and disease.

EMOTIONAL BODY ISSUES

A medical perspective from Jeff Migdow, M.D.

OUR EMOTIONS ARE like flowing water, constantly in motion. When we are thrown off emotionally, it's like a raging river where everything is thrown off course and anything can happen. Emotional body imbalance may lead to feelings of anger, resentment, betrayal, sadness, jealousy, grief, pain—very intense emotions that are difficult to shake off. Like a mad dog biting at our sleeve, our emotions grab on and hang on for dear life. Even the most rational argument can't get someone to drop their emotional upset. It's usually time that heals our emotional body. Sometimes we hold on to a particular emotion for years after the catalyzing event. Emotions are healthy and natural; it's the holding on long after the event has passed that leads to the disease of emotional imbalance and symptoms like agitation, abusing others or ourselves, severe digestive problems, menstrual difficulties, low back pain, and mental upset.

When the water element becomes agitated, it drives the subtler mental body in all directions. People who are emotionally distraught have the hardest time thinking clearly, and they lose the ability to connect with their intuition and find a solution to rebalance the emotional body. The tools for this body—such as clear communication, expression through music such as singing and drumming, or a good cry with someone we trust—help calm the troubled waters and bring us to a calmer emotional state, which allows the body to relax, the mind to calm down, and our intuition to emerge, giving us creative solutions to our problem and reminding us that the answers are within to find peace and health.

Depression

Depression is a widespread phenomenon in our society. Depression is the process of being so overwhelmed emotionally that we shut down our emotional body and become numb to our feelings, leading to a deeply empty hopeless, helpless state. Almost all of us have experienced this at one time or another, usually due to a loss or disappointment in life. We then over time overcome the depression and come back to ourselves. However, many of us, after multiple disappointments and losses, go into a more permanent shutdown state, which leads to more chronic depression. Once the depression lasts over a few weeks, the other bodies also become affected. The mind loses its sharpness and clarity and begins to dwell on negative, self-destructive thinking. We begin to obsess more about what we've lost, and we become stuck in the past. Our physical body becomes fatigued and unsteady; unable to sleep, we become more exhausted. As we move less, aches and pains occur, and our diet falls apart as we lose the motivation to eat in a healthy way, leading to digestive and hormonal disorders and a weakened immune system. Finally, as we lose our hope and feel helpless, our spiritual body becomes disconnected from Spirit, and we feel spiritually lost. This is a true crisis in living, as all the bodies have become weakened and disconnected.

Sleep-evaluation research reports that between 2–6 percent of the general population in the United States and Europe are depressed.[19] This would be between 6–18 million people in the United States—a huge number of people at any given time feeling the darkness of helplessness, hopelessness, lack of mental clarity, and loss of physical vitality and spiritual connection.

The rate of depression is higher in special groups. For example, the Agency for Healthcare Research reports that in pregnant woman, the incidence of depression is between 8.5–11 percent during pregnancy and 2.9–6.5 percent during the first year after delivery.[20] Other studies have shown the percentage of people with depression who have multiple sclerosis, chronic lung disease, cancer, and chronic heart disease are all higher than the national average. Thus, physical body disease itself can lead to or compound emotional body depression.

Finally, it was shown in a study that approximately 26 percent of Americans between the ages of 17–39 suffer from some form of depression, ranging from a major depressive episode to chronic depression.[21] This is the time when we are breaking away from our parents and the womb of the home and moving into a more independent, responsible life, making major decisions about education, profession, family, and children that will affect the rest of our lives and ranging into the time when the results of these decisions manifest in terms of finances, lifestyle, relationships, marriage partner, and raising

19   An example is a study done in 1999 by Ohayon, Priest, Guilleminault, and Caulet that shows how in their particular area the depression rate was 4.3 percent, and that in the United Kingdom the rate was 4.7 percent (published in the United Kingdom in *Biological Psychiatry* 1999, 45: 300–7).

20   See http://www.uptodate.com/patients/content/topic.do?topicKey=~KSjEZMzYAvxzi6.

21   This study was done between 1988 and 1994 by B. S. Jonas, D. Brody, M. Roper, and W. E. Narrow for the Centers for Disease Control and Prevention in Hyattsville, MD.

our children and building our homes and futures. These results and other comparable studies and estimates show that our society does not prepare us for this important time in our lives or give us much support. We often feel alone, on our own, cast into the big world like a boat without a rudder, as we have few social systems to help us cope with the huge changes that occur between the ages of 16 and 40. This is where the 4 Body Fit tools are so important for our lives and development, as they allow us to find ways in our day-to-day life to empower us to get through these years and the later years in a much more balanced, clear, connected, vital, and healthy way. This creates a feeling of both inner power and freedom that leads us to build relationships and ties to other people who are also doing the work to empower themselves, creating groups of people and communities of connection through yoga classes, meditation retreats, empowerment workshops, drumming circles, sweat lodge groups, and all the connections that are springing up from the experience of individuals using tools to help them help themselves live a fuller, freer life.

Disease of the Emotional Body: A Case Study

A forty-eight-year-old woman whom I had seen years before came to see me after the winter holidays to help her with headaches, fatigue, difficulty sleeping, and lack of appetite. She was wondering if it might be a thyroid disease or some dietary problem. She had been experiencing these symptoms for the past two months.

We talked for a while, and I felt she was not only fatigued but sad. I mentioned this and asked her if she had experienced any recent losses. She started to cry and told me that she had lost a close female friend the previous spring and had gone through months of grieving but felt she had moved on. We agreed from her crying that she still was grieving inside and had begun to block it when she felt the pain was dragging on—that is, she hadn't let the emotional grief reaction run its natural course. I suggested that perhaps the holidays had reactivated the grief. She agreed with this, saying they had always spent the holidays together and that the sleeplessness and fatigue had begun a week prior to Christmas, and the headaches and eating problems had started right before New Year's.

We spoke about this relationship and how close a friend this woman had been, and what a deep emotional loss it was. After more crying and talking, she felt more herself and not so constricted. She realized that her symptoms weren't a physical problem but had stemmed from depression related to blocking the grief reaction. Depression is the blocking of a deep emotional reaction, which leads us to a deep, empty space. We decided to work on this level, and she began using tools to allow her emotions to release naturally. She spoke to the people close to her about how she was still grieving so that she would feel comfortable with allowing the emotions to run their course. She went back to her weekly chanting group (which she had stopped after her friend passed away) to help release the feelings through song. I also prescribed a homeopathic remedy to help grief flow more smoothly and a flower remedy to help her feel the deeper feelings that she had suppressed. When she returned the next month, she was still in a grief process, but it had lessened to the point that she felt more comfortable in her daily activities, was sleeping and eating better, and had more energy and no headaches.

She is a good example of what happens when we block the natural cycle of our emotions; like trying to dam up water, they spill out somewhere else, often manifesting in physical symptoms, mental agitation, or spiritual emptiness. By feeling our feelings more deeply and giving them the space to emerge, they actually are cleared more quickly, allowing the other bodies to balance and heal.

SELF-TEST TO DISCOVER THE CURRENT STATE OF YOUR EMOTIONAL BODY

The following questionnaire is designed to enable you to find your strengths and weaknesses in the emotional body. It is also beneficial for strengthening self-awareness, which is key in being able to objectively see yourself clearly and from there be able to create more openness, strength, and balance in your life.

Take time for each question, and answer in a way that feels truthful to you. If you have areas where you feel like you aren't being honest, know that these are the places in which you tend to fool yourself. Usually these are the areas that need the most work.

Give yourself 5 points for *always*, 4 for *often*, 3 for *sometimes*, 2 for *occasionally*, and 1 for *never*. Then add up your totals for each body to get the grand total. This will help you objectively see where you stand in this body. As you move through this book and take the tests for the other bodies, compare the totals to see where your imbalances lie. We suggest you do each of these questionnaires every one to two months to check your progress and give you time to reflect.

Questions	
Key: always (5 points), often (4), sometimes (3), occasionally (2), never (1)	
1. I dance and express my emotions through my body.	3
2. When emotions come up, I step back and take time to reflect on what I am feeling.	4
3. I feel fulfilled and appreciated.	4
4. I deal well with my and others' emotions.	3
5. I feel free to ask when I need love and caring.	3
6. I feel that my lifestyle supports my emotional needs.	3
7. I communicate my emotions clearly with my family, friends, and coworkers.	4
8. I allow myself to feel my emotions fully until they naturally release, such as through crying.	4

Tally your score by adding up the points that correspond to each of your answers, and jot it down in a notebook or journal. Although 40 is a perfect score, where you fall on the scale today is not as important as seeing your scores improve over time, both numerically and in relation to your other bodies. (You don't want one score to be off the charts, with others far behind, for example.) As you test all four bodies, you'll begin to see how you can bring more balance to your entire being. If, for example, you scored a 36 on your spiritual body test, and later realize that your physical body fitness is only a 14, you can use that information to bring those numbers onto a more equal plane, perhaps by meditating less and working out more.

Strengthening the Emotional Body

Rebuilding emotional intelligence establishes security and sanity. When we learn how to create space in our lives to feel emotions we can understand the intelligence of emotions as energy, not just feelings. This intelligence is far greater than any book intelligence because emotions are the essence of being human. We cannot escape them, deny them, numb them, or outsmart them. They will eventually catch up to us and make us look straight into the depths of our soul to grow, learn, love, and evolve as a spiritual and human being. The best way I learned to work with my emotions was understanding the chakra system, which helped me understand the blueprint of my life: what I am doing, why I am doing it, and how it is affecting me. I ask myself these three questions constantly to challenge, treat, and heal myself so I can change the unhealthy emotional patterns in my life that are creating my present and leading to my future.

These exercises will help you tune in to your emotions, release excess or pent-up emotions, and bring awareness to where your emotions are taking up space in your body and mind. These exercises will help you let go of the baggage of the past, old emotional patterns of bad habits that lead you to react, not act. And they will enable you to build and strengthen your core on an emotional level to regain stability and security in the present, which shapes your future.

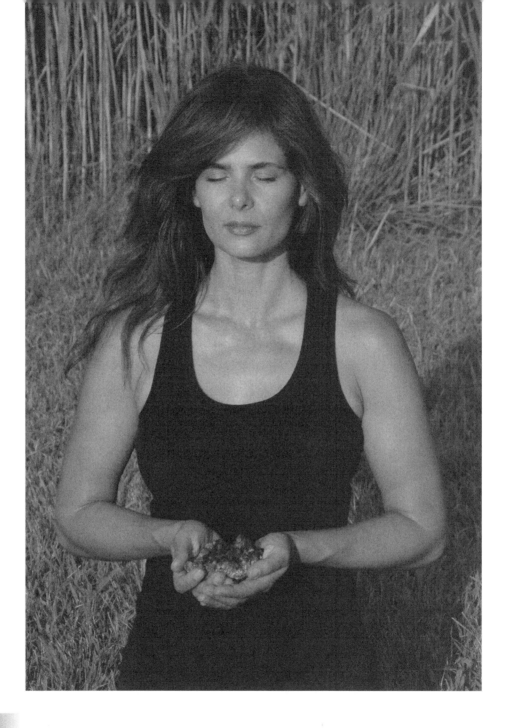

Holding crystals

AN INSIDE-OUT WORKOUT FOR
THE EMOTIONAL BODY

The following tools and exercises are practices to release and heal emotions and create flexibility and strength in the emotional body. I call them emotional core crunches, as they strengthen all eight muscles of the emotional body, connect you to your emotional intelligence, and strengthen your energetic field.

Holding Crystals

As discussed in the mental body, holding or wearing a crystal has healing properties. Though it may seem very subtle, it is working on a very deep level, helping you cleanse, release, and heal.

Tourmaline, for example, has a high lithium content, which helps relax the nervous system, bringing calmness to the mental and emotional bodies. Tourmaline interacts with all of the seven major chakras to cleanse, clear, and maintain them. It is known to shamans all over the world as a powerful healing stone that helps release old patterns and wounds. It is known to release the victim within. This is a wonderful stone for depression and to balance mood swings. The most common colors of tourmaline are pink and green.

I wore a piece of watermelon tourmaline on my heart for years. I worked with girls aged five through thirteen who lived in a foster home in New Jersey. They had been brutally abused and taken from their homes for their own safety. I donated my services twice a week to help them deal with their abuse. Most were on antidepressants, violent, and overweight; their future did not look good. I taught them how to use yoga, breathwork, healing stones, exercise, massage, anger management (a baseball bat to a mattress), and diet to reprogram their nervous system to release the issues in their tissues and to take back their life. In three months, they were off drugs, more self-sufficient, exercising on their own, calm, and eating right. The foster care home did not understand how it happened so quickly.

I taught them prayer, faith, hope, anger management, and how to receive touch and take back their life. They were empowered and proud of it. They were relieved that someone they trusted had validated their pain, knew what it felt like, and did not think they were bad, crazy, or out of control. No one had told them how to deal with their pain, what had happened to them and why.

Being and sharing with the girls, I healed myself and my own issues—the victim of abuse within me. The day I left the foster home two years later, my watermelon tourmaline necklace broke in half. As my heart broke open, so did the stone.

When you explain to someone what they are doing, why they are doing it, and how it is affecting them, they receive knowledge about themselves. And if they choose to ignore this information, then they have made the choice to live with the consequences and remain a victim with a capital V. This is the boot camp in me, but it is what has saved my life.

Aromatherapy

Aromatherapy is the skilled use of essential oils. It dates back 5,000 years ago and was used by the Egyptians and Hindus. The holy men used frankincense to cleanse their holy places, and even Jesus Christ was blessed with frankincense and myrrh.

As we discussed in the mental body, essential oils are another great tool to help you not only heal but nurture yourself. It is an ancient secret that women passed down to each other for medical, holistic, aesthetic, and ritual purposes.

All essential oils are antibacterial, anticancerous, antifungal, antimicrobial, antiparasitic, antiviral, and antiseptic. Whether you use oils for massage, use on your pillowcases for relaxation, rub on to heal a scar or burn, or use them to disinfect your room, oils create a free radical space within us and our environment.

Essential oils' bioelectrical frequency is several times greater than the frequency of herbs, food, and even the human body. Essentials oils come from such sources as bark, resins, flowers, leaves, roots, fruits, and seeds. And because the DNA structure of these resources in nature are similar to the DNA of a human being's essence, they work naturally and holistically. The essence of nature reflects human life.

Out of all the five senses, our most primitive sense is smell. Because the nostrils are so close to the brain, smell influences our fight-or-flight response and our hormones, pheromones, and cellular memory. For instance, when you smell an odor, it can be pleasant or unpleasant, depending on your experience. You walk into your grandma's home and always smell chocolate chip cookies and the memories of making them with her. Every time you smell chocolate chip cookies or even see them, it will stimulate the brain and five senses, sending a message to the brain and cellular level of the emotions you were feeling at the time: warm, loving, fun, safe.

For someone who has been raped, it can work the opposite way. They remember the smell of the cologne or the hair product their abuser was wearing. When they smell this odor, it will bring up painful memories and even flashbacks of the event.

I know this was true for me. My abuser wore Old Spice, and every time I smelled it, I panicked. It put my fight-or-flight response on overload; deep terror crawled up my spine. Although it happened years ago, it was still embedded in my cellular makeup—a memory that was now embedded in my emotional body, which gave a signal to my brain/mental body to have negative thoughts and my physical body to become paralyzed by fear. I could never figure out why until I studied aromatherapy and healing work.

I wanted to erase these memories from my core like erasing a chalkboard. I was determined to do it, and I did. Through all the work on all four levels, I did it, and the last validation was this: I was traveling in Peru to visit Machu Picchu on my Goddess Sacred yearly tour with a group of women. The cab driver was wearing a cologne that smelled great to me. I am not a perfume or cologne fan, but this man was so good looking and his cologne was driving me crazy. My pheromones were heightened. I asked him to please tell me what he was wearing, and he said Old Spice. I just about died. I literally cried, for I knew I had truly erased the abuse from every cell of my being. All the work I have done to heal myself holistically and naturally was proven and validated.

In choosing an essential oil, the nose knows. The body's natural, native intelligence will tell you what it wants and what it is attracted to. You can create a blend for your daily ritual massage after your shower or bath and another for your perfume.

Massage Body Blend:
YOUR GODDESS BLEND

1. Use a carrier oil (a base oil to mix with your essential oils) such as almond, olive, or sunflower; use enough to almost fill a four- to eight-ounce bottle.

2. Pick the essential oils you would like to use for your blend; three to five essential oils for a four- to eight-ounce bottle of carrier oil is enough.

3. Place fifteen drops total inside your carrier oil bottle, using all three to five essential oils. You can be your own scientist: smell the oils with each other

as you go, do not just put them in and mix. Some oils have a stronger smell than others and will mask them if you are not careful. Again, the nose knows what it will like; do this slowly and carefully.

4. Once you blend them all together, shake the bottle and store in a warm, dark place when not using.

5. Rub on your body after every bath and shower.

Perfume:

GODDESS MAGIC THAT WILL DRIVE YOUR PARTNER CRAZY

I always leave my scent everywhere: when I am gone, I place my oil blend in a card on the bed and leave my oils on the pillowcases and even my underwear. Do not think he does not smell me everywhere while I am gone. My goddess blend will bring up very intimate memories, which will keep his mind in the right place. They say a man thinks about sex an average of every thirty seconds to a minute; would you *not* have him thinking of you? It's the magic and mystery of the goddess that always keeps them guessing and begging for more. Do remember that smell is the most primitive sense for men.

When you work with your pheromones, your perfume works for you. Your personal perfume will put out a smell that will drive people crazy. Scent is a very primitive yet sensual dance—one your partner will never forget. Try this and see for yourself!

1. Pick what you are most attracted to; you can pick one, two, or three oils. I use patchouli, frankincense, and amber; they all offset each other, creating an earthy yet sweet smell.

2. No need for carrier oil: place the oil directly on skin (this is called a neat application). Put on erogenous zones—behind knees, neck, wrists, pelvis.

3. Since your prana, your life force, puts off heat, it penetrates the oils and leaves a lofting smell in the air others will never forget.

Benefits:
- Excellent for moisturizing your skin.
- Strengthens the immune system.
- Relaxing.
- Releases pent-up emotions.

- Reprograms the nervous system's fight-or-flight response.

- Brings oxygen to the cells.

- Kills bacteria.

- Strengthens and cleans your energetic auric field.

- Wonderfully sensual.

- Balances hormones.

Singing/Chanting

As we discussed in the spiritual body, singing a meaningful song connects your heart to the heart of the universe. Singing connects us to our feelings and allows us to feel more comfortable and confident expressing ourselves and working with the water element within all of us. It is as if you were talking and praying to God, or Spirit, in another way.

When we chant from our heart to Goddess, God, or Nature, our deeper emotions of love and longing emerge. These emotions are core feelings that our other emotions ride on. The love feelings bring out emotions of joy and compassion, while the longing feelings bring up sadness and grief.

Benefits:

When we express these feelings fully, they flow through us and are released, leaving us feeling fresh, new, and open. This creates space for other emotions, such as anger, resentment, and sadness, to be felt and expressed more freely. Also, the words of the chanting—be they yogic, Native American, English, or any language—carry spiritual vibrations that open the heart center and emotions more fully.

Bathing

Connecting to the water element is nurturing, replenishing, cleansing, and purifying. Water is the blood of Mother Earth. Water is a conductor of energy, which vibrates the cells of our being and brings nutrients to the cells. Where there is friction within you, call the element of water to create flow and fluidity and to walk the path of least resistance.

We drink water to cleanse the toxins from our system internally, and when we bath or shower, we also cleanse externally unseen toxins in our energetic field and aura.

Next time you come across a natural spring, river, ocean, or lake, bless yourself with the water and give thanks for its life force, for without water we cannot survive. With our natural water supply being in a state of extinction, be aware of the water element in your life.

Bathing is a wonderful way to relax and nurture the water element of emotions. I take a bath weekly or after every workshop with sea salt and my oils to soften my skin, cleanse my aura and energetic field, and get more in tune with my emotions and intuition. Remember: water creates electricity and opens our third eye to flow with our psychic abilities.

While taking a shower in the morning, visualize all the toxins you have taken on in your energetic body and your emotional body spiraling down the drain from head to toe. Next time you are at the beach, honor the goddess of sea and water, Yemaya, by cleansing and basking yourself in her beauty and natural waters.

Chakra-Balancing Meditations

As I discussed earlier in the spiritual body, each part of the body, each chakra, resonates with a sound, vibration, sensation, and frequency. While you sit and meditate, sing the sounds out loud—feel the movement of the sound through *all* your bodies. Using all of your senses, gauge what the color of the chakra smells like, feels like, tastes like, looks like, and sounds like as it moves in and out of your body and through your mouth.

Each chakra has a female and male sound (see chart on next page). The front of the body is receptive to the energy of the universe—the female aspects, while the back of the body is the will center, putting our energy out to the universe—the male aspects. The female sounds are sung once and long, and the male sounds are sung three times in a row. As you start from the root chakra up to the crown, first start off with the female sound, then remain in silence for a brief moment before singing the male sounds. Repeat for each chakra. This is a wonderful exercise of expression and learning how to work with your emotions and energy on a deeper, more intuitive level.

Can you sense if your chakras and parts of your body are open, closed, or even working and vibrating to their full potential?

Chakra	Female Sounds	Male Sounds
Root	O	Lam, Lam, Lam
Sexual	OO	Vam, Vam, Vam
Solar Plexus	AH	Ram, Ram, Ram
Heart	AY	Yam, Yam, Yam
Throat	EE	Hum, Hum, Hum
Third Eye	MM	Om
Crown	Silence	Ommmmm

Emotional Release Work

Learn to move and work with your emotions. Find what is appropriate for your emotions, such as getting out your rage and anger by beating a punching bag with a bat, or sitting under a tree and being in a state of joy. You must learn how to validate and give yourself permission to feel; in order to do this, you must create the space for that emotion in your life. Do not fear them; become one with them—they are a part of you and the human essence. Also remember that no one else can feel your pain but you. It is yours, and you need to own it, not project it because you are uncomfortable with it. Stop trying to analyze them; emotions are not in your head but in your heart.

Drumming

Drumming has been used since the beginning of humanity for the purpose of not only communication but also emotional expression. The playing of the drum from the heart allows deep emotions to be felt, expressed, and released. This tool is especially effective in a group where people take turns drumming; thus all are getting the benefits both while drumming and dancing to the beat. Women were known to be the first drummers, and today there are many women's drumming circles all over the world. In many native cultures, the drum represents Mother Earth's heartbeat and our heartbeat working as one. The beat of the drum was used in birthing ceremonies to help women with contractions. The drum is the primal sound of the lower part of the body—the animalistic and primitive parts of us. The drum dates back before written language to 40,000 BC and was used by the high priestesses in healing ceremonies to raise the vibrations of lower energies, ward off evil spirits such disease, and speak to other tribes from afar.

Drumming also brings balance to the right and left hemispheres of the brain. The drum synchronizes our alpha and beta brain waves, creating a trancelike state that brings heightened awareness, tapping into the higher consciousness of our being.

The sound of the drum represents the heartbeat of Mother Earth and our heart connecting as one. Do you know your own rhythm and flow (dancing to the beat of your own drum, as they say), or do you follow the crowd?

Benefits:

Since the drum is nonverbal, we can go more deeply into the primal emotions of bliss, rage, and deep pain, releasing them through the beat of the drum.

Dancing

In many native cultures, the dance symbolizes the dance of life. We must be flexible yet strong, graceful yet have the stamina to move through life. Like drumming, dancing is an ancient ritual and tool for the release of deep emotion. In the process of free dancing, we come in touch with any emotion that is under the surface at that moment. It is then felt, expressed, and released, allowing new feelings to emerge. Combined with drumming and chanting, as is done in Native American and Eastern Indian ceremonies, it is a wonderful way to access and express deep emotions in a group setting.

Dance is a ritual that helps us connect with Mother Earth under our feet and rejoice in Father Sky, our Great Spirit, giving thanks for what we have. Dances are rituals that help us call in the spirits above and below for guidance and gratitude. When we allow ourselves the freedom of movement in our bodies, we can channel whatever emotion we need to. Natives do not intellectualize their emotions, they work through them with their bodies. The young boys learn to work with fire to understand their anger and primitive need for control, which can burn them in more ways then one. Power yoga was a practice for young men to harness the fire of their emotions and hormones; now it is a common practice for all yogis in the United States, but no one really asks why. The natives taught me how to work with my emotions through physical activity.

I would walk until I would just about drop. In the process of walking, I would take short breaths, putting my body in a constant state of fight-or-flight, my mind was unable to focus, and when I felt I could go no longer, I dropped to my knees, dug a hole in the ground, screamed into it, and then covered the hole, burying it to give it all to Mother Earth to help heal. With every scream, I felt how wonderful it was to release. Instead of taking emotions out on others and reacting, we must learn to channel our emotions so that we do not become violent with ourselves or others. It is not good or bad energy, it is energy to the universe. You will not hurt the earth by giving it away, but you will hurt yourself, others, and the planet if you continue to hold back—and we wonder why people just pick up a gun and start shooting others. We are pressure cookers ready to blow! You can only simmer so long before you boil over.

This balance is greatly put into effect in the laws of the universe and natural rhythm and flow of Mother Earth. Volcanoes, tsunamis, floods, fires—all of which have been happening in our lifetime—are all expressions of Mother Earth's anger, toxins, and emotional overload of energy. If we are all one and all connected, then we have to know that our planet is a reflection of our own emotional overload.

Mother Earth has fires to clean out a forest, volcanoes to refertilize the earth, and diseases to kill the animal and plant kingdom to create equilibrium, balance, and harmony within herself. It is her way of detoxifying herself through her elements; we must recognize that the balance of these elements within ourselves works the same way. When we suppress our emotions or fear we do not have enough love, money, or food—all things that Mother Earth provides for us—it leads to unconscious choices and unhealthy reactions.

BREATHING FOR THE EMOTIONAL BODY

Breath is the food that revitalizes, reenergizes, and recycles our emotions to reprogram, build, and maintain a healthy emotional body. The exercises below greatly affect the adrenal glands, immune system, and nervous system, all of which are the major components to healing the energetic blueprint to release you from addiction, abuse, weight loss, eating disorders, and depression. If you continue to do these exercises every day, which should only take you up to twenty minutes, you will heal in three months. The hard part is then maintaining and making it a daily practice for the rest of your life.

Warning: If you choose not to make this commitment of twenty minutes a day to your well-being, then you must live with the consequences and realize you are creating your own pain, your own reality. As I discussed earlier in the mental body, not enough serotonin in the brain is the major cause of many illnesses. These exercises will release serotonin at a high rate and are a natural way of helping you balance and come into alignment with your true, authentic, healthy self.

The Importance of Breath

The breath is the energetic food that feeds the emotional body. Without it, we become toxic, overreactive, irritable, depressed. Breathing releases serotonin into the brain, and when you go back to the mental body, not enough serotonin in the brain is the major cause of depression, addiction, obesity, and many other diseases. The quality of our breathing is directly related to our quality of life.

Most people only use a quarter of their lung capacity. Proper breathing techniques teach you to expand your lung capacity, feel your emotions, and experience the strength to let go.

The breath is the rhythm and flow of our life force. Breath gives life to all living things. Deep breathing helps to cleanse and nourish the body and mind. The breath we take in feeds every cell of our being. The breath we exhale removes toxins from the bloodstream and organs.

The breath is the first thing to enter the body when we are born and the last to leave when we die. The more naturally we can breathe and move, the more energized we become. As the body, mind, and spirit begin to function together, we feel more alive and refreshed.

Most people do not use their full lung capacity on a physical level because they have not been taught how to breathe properly. In the yogic world it is called pranayama, breath control. The practice of breathing connects us to the life force that feeds us. On the emotional level, people do not breathe into their lungs and heart because it shifts energy and consciousness, therefore bringing up deep emotions. Wherever there is no breath, the organs, glands, and systems of that area do not receive nutrients to the cells, thereby creating cancer, heart disease, thyroid problems, and much more. If you only breathe short, quick breaths into the lower part of your body, how do the other parts of your body receive oxygen? Just as athletes will go to higher altitudes (mountains) to train in order to expand their lung capacity, so must we also climb that mountain on a spiritual and emotional level to train our energetic bodies.

Spiritually, the breath allows us to tap into our intuition, our holistic intelligence and connection to Spirit. Mentally, the breath brings balance to the left and right hemispheres of the brain. The breath releases serotonin into the brain to feel relaxed and stress free. And as we now know, too little serotonin in the brain is the major cause of addiction, depression, and weight gain. Emotionally, the breath allows us to release pent-up emotions and issues stored in our tissues from past hurts and pains. Physically, the breath brings more oxygen into our body, and oxygen burns fat in the simplest form and feeds the cells of our body, preventing and healing disease and dis-ease in the body.

In summary, the breath can provide an abundance of energy to rejuvenate, delay the aging process, burn fat, speed metabolism, clear the mind, focus on healthy thoughts, reprogram cells, erase tension and anxiety, balance right and left hemispheres of the brain, and release pent-up emotions.

Benefits of deepening your practice of breathing exercises:

- Awaken emotional intelligence and the body's native intelligence.
- Gain a strong sense of self.
- Improve range of motion and emotion.
- Increase flexibility.
- Balance the emotions.
- Feel and heal.

- Learn the strength to let go.

- Relieve stress.

- Release cellular memory.

Ha Breath
THE BREATH OF RELEASE

1. Start in a standing position, your feet in a squat or straddle position. Lift your arms straight over your head, towards the sky, and take a deep inhale through your nostrils.

2. Squat down and shout a big *Ha* forcefully at the same time.

3. Pull your arms down and pull universal energy into your belly (solar plexus). Repeat ten times.

4. Still in standing position, drop your arms to your sides, and using the ha breath, squat and pull Mother Earth energy into your belly (solar plexus). Repeat ten times.

5. Still in standing position, your feet hip-width apart, bring your arms forward and pulling your arms in toward your belly (solar plexus) arms at the side of your waist, uniting both universal forces—Father Sky and Mother Earth.

Benefits:

The ha breath is wonderful to let go of stress and pent-up emotions. Use this breath to exert your energy, especially when using weights in your workout or when you have the need to let go or desire an energy boost. The ha breath will:

- Improve digestion.

- Strengthen internal organs.

- Relieve constipation.

- Create a feeling of being grounded and centered.

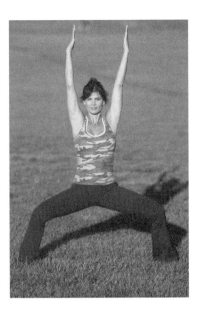

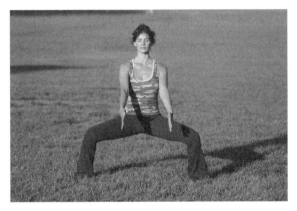

 *Ha breath*

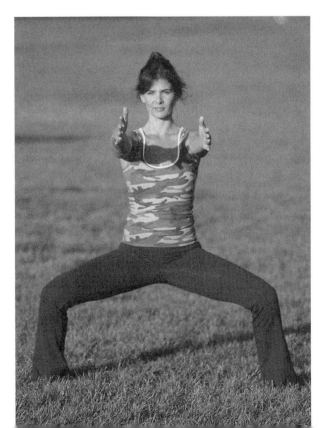

Water/Ocean Breath
SANSKRIT NAME: UJJAYI

Ujjayi, or natural breath, is the element of water and emotions. It is the breath of natural flow and rhythm of breathing, which actually sounds like the ocean. To breathe fully in your heart and lungs, you must understand how your breath works first. Most of us only use a quarter of our lung capacity and breathe from the belly button down, which actually puts our nervous system's fight-or-flight response in reactive overload. However, when you learn to breathe into your heart and lungs, you reprogram your nervous system, therefore quieting the mind, opening the heart, and relaxing the body. Serotonin is naturally released, and you feel at peace.

To tune in and listen to sound of your own breath, place your hands over your ears and breath in and out of your nostrils only. Your breath will sound like the ocean and as if you placed a conch shell up to your ear.

How to Breathe Properly

1. Come into a seated position with spine erect.

2. Place your palm in front of your face as if you are holding a mirror, and exhale out through your mouth, as if you are going to fog up that mirror. Hear the wispiness and feel the pressure of the exhale.

3. Breath in the back of your throat.

4. Repeat the same directions, but this time exhale through your nostrils only.

5. Hear the wispiness again and feel the pressure of the exhale breath in the back of your throat. This wispiness makes the sound of the ocean.

6. Now concentrate on the inhale breath being just as strong as the exhale breath.

7. Inhale and take a slow, long, and deep breath through your nostrils into your throat, expanding your chest and filling your lungs.

As you inhale, the breath moves upward from the pelvis to the belly, heart, and lungs like a wave breaking gently on the shore.

Lying Down Variation

1. Lay on the floor.

2. Place a pillow under your diagraphm (where your bra strap is). This pillow will help lift your rib cage, heart, and diagraphm up towards the sky.

3. Chin lifts up towards the sky and throat is open.

4. Arms should be six inches away from your body with palms open.

5. Breathe in and out of nostrils only.

6. Fill your pelvis, belly, heart, and lungs with your breath.

It will not be easy at first, but practice expanding your ribs like a gills of a fish, allowing more breath and oxygen to fill every ounce of your being. Visualize a wave as your breath fills up the pelvis, belly, heart, and lungs, and exhale all the toxins out of your body through your nostrils only.

All of these benefits lead to a faster metabolism, stronger immune system, ability to burn fat at a faster rate, and help prevent heart and respiratory diseases.

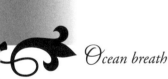 *Ocean breath*

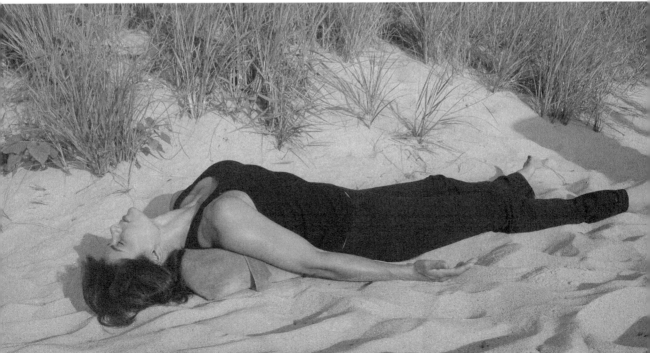

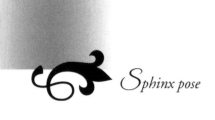

Sphinx pose

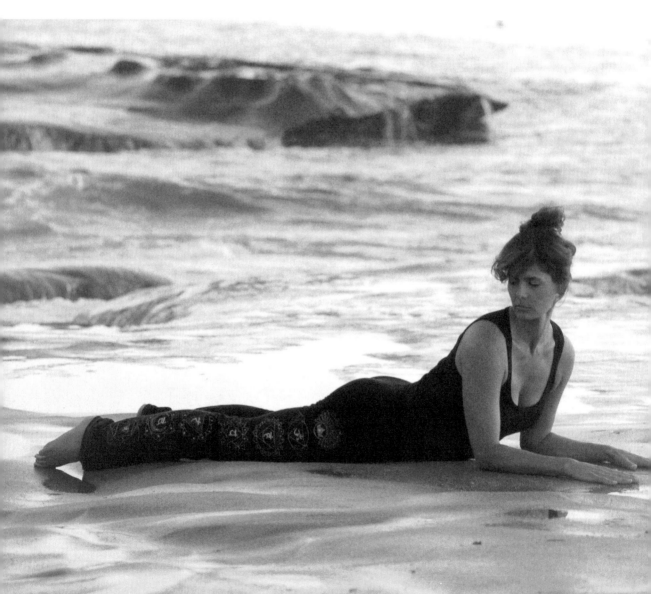

YOGA POSES FOR THE EMOTIONAL BODY

Yoga is the science and practice of self: self-awareness, self-acceptance, and self-love. Each posture will reflect your weaknesses and strengths. Are you able to go into pain or do you run from pain? Breathe, have patience, and know that yoga is not about being flexible but being in the present moment so that you can stop, look, listen, and feel what is going on within. It is about intention, not perfection. The physical body will always benefit from what you do internally first and work its way out to the external.

Sphinx/Protection
SANSKRIT NAME: ARDHA BHUJANGASANA

The sphinx is a female temple guardian. She was placed in front of many architectural structures such as royal tombs or religious temples to protect them. She has the body of a lioness and a human head.

Steady and simple, this pose allows complete relaxation to occur and the wisdom of Spirit to come through. The head stands observant yet focused, the spine lengthens as the fire of passion and compassion awakens within, and the body holds firm and wields her power—peaceful yet fierce. Do you stand in power? Do you know how to protect yourself?

Entry and Holding Posture

1. Lie on your belly on the floor with your arms bent, elbows directly underneath your shoulders on the floor, forearms and palms shoulder-width apart. Spread the fingers and press into ground, holding firm—this reprograms the nervous system.

2. Do not engage the buttocks; feel the pelvis drop deeper into the earth with each breath.

3. Keep the crown of the head lifted and shoulders down and away from the ears.

4. Feel the lower back, adrenals, kidneys, and ovaries all being engaged.

Looking forward, hold up to 15–30 seconds—about five big breaths through the nostrils only. Looking over your right shoulder, hold for up to 15–30 seconds. Repeat, looking over your left shoulder.

Benefits and Systems Being Treated, Challenged, and Healed:
- Strengthens and lengthens the spine.
- Compresses adrenals, releasing serotonin to the brain.
- Compresses the ovaries, bringing balance to hormones.
- Compresses the thymus, strengthening the immune system.
- Compresses the kidney, flushing toxins and pent-up emotions.
- Calms the nervous system—great for insomnia or depression.

Precautions and Contraindications:
- Back injury

Cobra Pose
Sanskrit Name: Bhujangasana

The cobra always has its eyes open. The crown and eyes lift to see, and the heart opens to new perspectives and transformation. The head rises with an awareness of its surroundings. The heart opens, and core strength is found. As the pelvis pushes down, a surge of power lengthens the spine. The cobra sheds its skin to grow. Are you able to shed the skin of self-doubt and turn your weaknesses into strengths? What do you need to shed? Are you able to rise up to defend your path and beliefs?

Entry and Holding Posture
1. Lay on your belly, feet together, third eye on the floor.
2. Place your hands, palms down, next to your ribs so that fingers are at the bra line. Spread your fingers and keep elbows tucked close to your sides.
3. Lift up through the crown, using your back muscles, keeping your shoulders down and back, away from your ears.
4. While your back muscles are engaged, you should be able to lift your hands one to two inches off the floor.

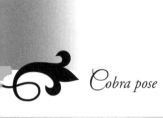

Cobra pose

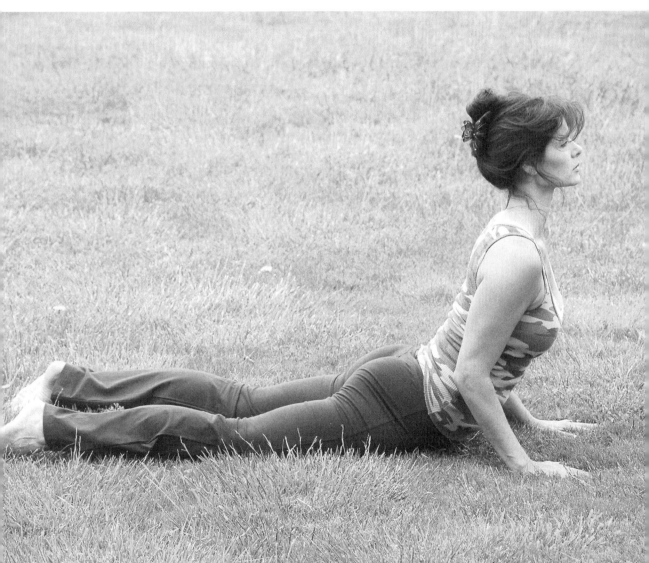

5. Place your hands back on the floor, next to the bra line, fingers spread. The middle fingers should be pointing straight ahead.

6. Press into your palms, lifting through your crown and opening your heart until you come approximately three-fourths of the way up, if you can. (Otherwise, you can raise up to a height that your own ability level will comfortably allow.) Engage the buttocks, keep shoulders down and pulled back, and open the heart.

7. Feel the squeeze on all your back muscles as they are engaged to support you.

8. Take five big breaths in and out through nostrils only, holding the posture for at least thirty seconds.

9. Release and relax, coming out of the posture.

10. Breathe and receive, feeling and allowing new openings of prana flow.

Repeat two or three times.

Benefits and Systems Being Treated, Challenged, and Healed:
- Tones ovaries and uterus.
- Compresses the adrenal glands, releasing serotonin.
- Compresses the kidneys, releasing grief.
- Strengthens lungs and facilitates deeper breathing.
- Reprograms the nervous system's fight-or-flight response.
- Releases tension and anxiety.
- Improves blood circulation.
- Improves spinal flexibility and back strength.
- Revitalizes adrenals.
- Strengthens immune system.

Precautions and Contraindications:

- Low back pain or weak back muscles should start with modified positions of the cobra.

- Pregnancy.

- High blood pressure.

- Heart disease.

- Stroke.

Boat Pose/Direction
NAVASANA

The boat must follow its course to reach its destination. The open heart lightens the load. The stomach pushes down and the legs extend, maintaining balance. The arms and head lift to see. The boat arrives at its destination when it is free to sail. Are you able to trust and let go and let God lead you to your destiny? Do you know how to let your sails down and enjoy the journey of life, or do you constantly try to control it? Is your boat set on course toward your desires? Are you ready to sail?

Entry and Holding Posture

While you are doing this pose, find a stationary focal point ten to twenty feet in front of you and do not take your eyes off it.

1. Lie on your belly with your arms near your sides, your palms down, and your legs approximately hip-width apart, with your chin on the floor.

2. Press into your pelvis while you engage your buttocks, back, and hamstrings.

3. Lift and lengthen through your arms and legs simultaneously.

4. Open the heart at the same time by keeping shoulders down and back and reaching through the chest.

5. Lift through the crown of your head, looking out onto the horizon.

6. Take in nice, big belly breaths, breathing in and out through your nostrils only, five to ten times.

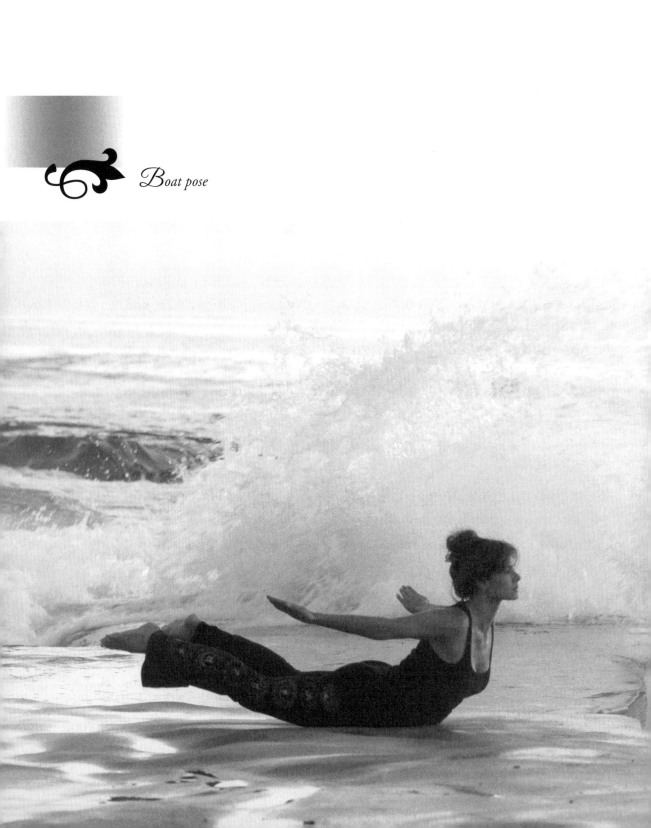

Boat pose

7. Release and slowly come out of the posture.

8. Lie on your stomach and breathe, receiving the prana that renews and rejuvenates your body.

Repeat two to three times.

ARM VARIATIONS:

1. Extend your arms out in front of your gaze, palms facing each other to set your course.

2. Bring your arms back behind you, interlacing the fingers, lengthening and lifting your clasped hands to set sail.

Benefits and Systems Being Treated, Challenged, and Healed:

• Irrigates kidneys with fresh blood supply, promoting elimination of toxins.

• Nourishes ovaries and uterus with fresh blood supply.

• Tones abdomen.

• Strengthens lungs and facilitates deeper breathing.

• Improves blood circulation.

• Increases body heat.

• Energizes entire body.

• Revitalizes entire endocrine system, especially adrenals and pancreas.

• Builds self-confidence.

• Strengthens buttocks, hamstrings, calves, abdomen, trapezoids, deltoids, heart, triceps, and upper, middle, and lower back.

• Promotes focus.

• Strengthens and relaxes the nervous system, releases serotonin into brain.

• Compresses the thymus, strengthening the immune system.

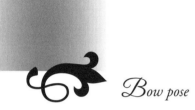

Bow pose

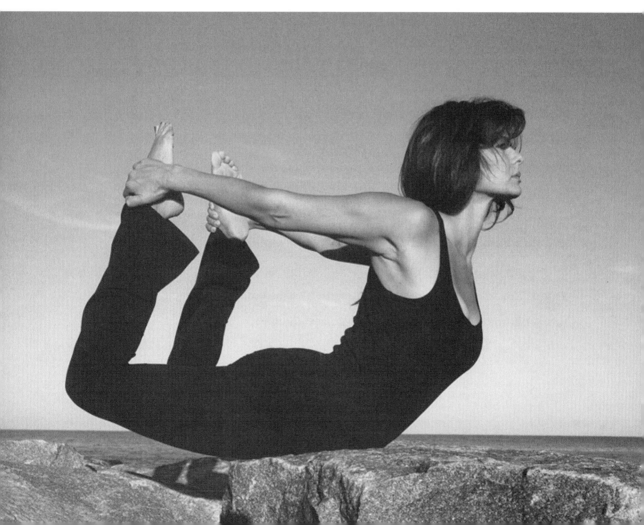

Precautions and Contraindications:

- Insure proper warmups before attempting the boat (i.e., cat/dog, sunbird, sphinx, and cobra).

- If you have weak back muscles, go easy.

- Pregnancy (after third month).

- Recent abdominal surgery or abdominal inflammation.

- Recent or chronic back injury or inflammation.

Bow Pose/Duality
Sanskrit name: Dhanurasana

The bow is both a weapon for protection and tool used to obtain food. The bow requires strength to pull, flexibility to bend, and wisdom to know when to let go—the balance of push and pull. What is your target in life? Do you know how to go after what you desire? Are you focused enough to get it?

Entry and Holding Posture

1. Lie facedown on your abdomen, forehead to floor and hands by your side.

2. With your legs about hip-width apart, bend your knees and bring your feet close to your buttocks. Grasp your legs at the ankles or feet, one at a time.

3. Inhale and press your feet into your hands, lifting your knees off the floor, toes pointed upwards, and lengthening your spine, and rise up, squeezing your shoulder blades and opening your heart.

4. Lift up through the crown of your head and find a focal point.

5. Find a balance between ease and effort. Focus on keeping the spine long and evenly arched instead of trying to lift up high.

6. Slowly relax body to start position.

Hold up to 15–30 seconds—about five big breaths through the nostrils only. Repeat two to three times.

Benefits and Systems Being Treated, Challenged, and Healed:

- Stretches the entire front of the body, ankles, thighs, groin, abdomen, chest, throat, and deep hip flexors.

- Strengthens the back muscles.

- Improves posture.

- Stimulates the organs of the abdomen and neck.

- Massages the abdomen and stimulates the digestive system.

- Creates fire in the belly, speeding up metabolism.

- Stimulates reproductive organs, including the kidneys and adrenal glands.

- Compresses the thymus, strengthening the immune system.

Precautions and Contraindications:

- Those with low back pain, neck pain, or shoulder injury should begin with half bow, one leg at a time.

- Should be avoided during pregnancy.

- Contraindicated for those with recent abdominal surgery, high blood pressure, heart disease, or stroke.

Camel/Endurance
Sanskrit name: Ustrasana

The camel has the durability to overcome harsh conditions. The legs' strength carries the weight of the body. The heart opens, and oxygen fuels the body. The spine arches from the tailbone to the head, where stamina is stored. The camel carries what it needs within itself. Can you endure life's challenges?

Entry and Holding Posture

1. Kneel on the floor with your knees hip-width apart and thighs perpendicular to the floor.

2. Rotate your thighs inward slightly, narrow your hip points, and firm but don't harden your buttocks. Imagine that you're drawing your sitting bones up, into your torso. Keep your outer hips as soft as possible.

3. Press your shins and the tops of your feet firmly into floor.

4. Rest your hands on the back of your pelvis, bases of the palms on the tops of the buttocks, fingers pointing down. Use your hands to spread the back pelvis and lengthen it down through your tailbone. Then lightly firm the tail forward, toward the pubis. Make sure that your groin doesn't "puff" forward; to prevent this, press your front thighs back, countering the forward action of your tail. Inhale and lift your heart by pressing the shoulder blades against your back ribs.

5. Now lean back against the firmness of the tailbone and shoulder blades. For the time being, keep your head up, chin near the sternum and hands on the pelvis.

6. If you need to, tilt the thighs back a little and minimally twist to one side to get one hand on the same-side foot. Then press your thighs back to perpendicular, turn your torso back to neutral, and touch the second hand to its foot. If you're not able to touch your feet without compressing your lower back, turn your toes under and elevate your heels.

7. Release the front ribs and lift the front of the pelvis up, toward the ribs. Then lift the lower back ribs away from the pelvis to keep the lower spine as long as possible. Press your palms firmly against your soles (or heels),

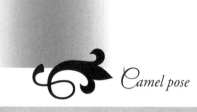

Camel pose

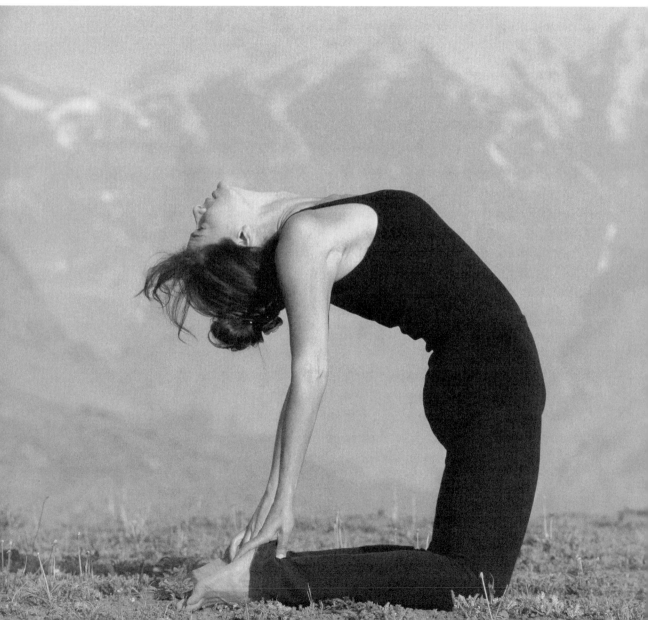

with the bases of the palms on the heels and the fingers pointing toward the toes. Turn your arms outwardly so the elbow creases face forward, without squeezing the shoulder blades together. You can keep your neck in a relatively neutral position, neither flexed nor extended, or drop your head back, but be careful not to strain your neck and harden your throat.

8. To exit, bring your hands onto the front of your pelvis at the hip points. Inhale and lift the head and torso up by pushing the hip points down toward the floor. If your head is back, lead with your heart to come up, not by jutting the chin toward the ceiling and leading with your forehead. Rest in child's pose for a few breaths.

Hold up to 15–30 seconds—about five big breaths through the nostrils only. Repeat two or three times.

Benefits and Systems Being Treated, Challenged, and Healed:
- Opens and engages the throat, the thyroid, and parathyroid.
- Opens the muscles of respiration for fuller breath (opens chest).
- Activates the thymus, strengthening the immune system, adrenals, and thymus.
- Good for breast cancer support.
- Stretches the entire front of the body, the ankles, thighs, groin, abdomen, chest, and throat.
- Stretches the deep hip flexors.
- Strengthens back muscles.
- Improves posture.
- Stimulates the organs of the abdomen and neck.
- Releases anger.
- Teaches compassion for self.
- Opens the diaphragm for fuller breathing.
- Squeezes the adrenals and kidneys, sending in fresh blood flow and oxygen.

- Releases serotonin to the brain and relaxes the nervous system's fight-or-flight response.

- Strengthens your core physically and emotionally.

Precautions and Contraindications:

- Weak back or neck muscles.

- Neck pain or injury, high blood pressure, heart disease, hypothyroid, or stroke.

- Low back or knee pain should use modifications.

- Migraines.

- Insomnia.

Modifications:

- Hands on the hips or lower back and slowly bend backwards.

- Front of the body against a wall.

- Hands on the heels or blocks with the toes tucked under.

Wheel/The Rainbow
SANSKRIT NAME: CHAKRASANA

The feet firmly press into the earth, the arms lift the head and heart, the spine arches, the heart reaches up toward Spirit, and the throat opens. The hips lift with power and purpose and release emotions. The endurance and stamina of the mind and heart are challenged to lengthen and strengthen.

Completely opening up takes strength, determination, and focus. Spirit helps you to follow your intuition, speak your truth, open your heart, breathe into your power, let go, and create the space to be filled with life, love, and joy. Just as the rainbow is the bridge between earth and heaven, the wheel is the bridge between mind, body, and spirit. Are your mind, body, and spirit connected?

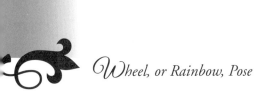

Wheel, or Rainbow, Pose

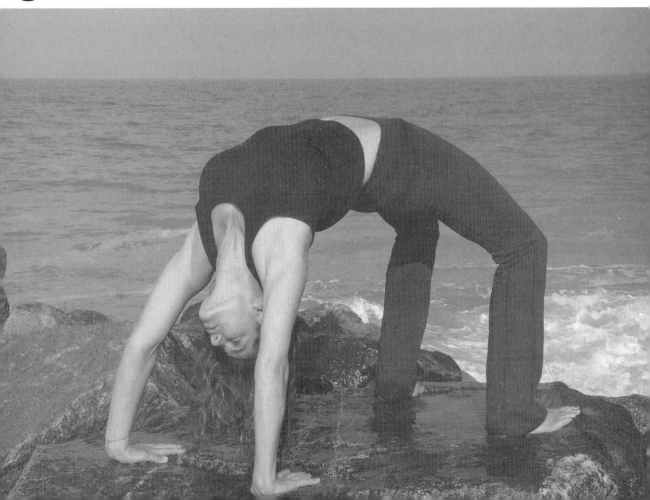

Entry and Holding Posture

1. Lying on your back, lengthen body, arms at your sides. Bend your knees and place the feet flat on the floor, a few inches from the buttocks, fingertips able to touch.

2. Place the hands flat on the ground and next to ears, shoulder-width apart.

3. Spread fingers wide, facing down toward the shoulders.

4. Lift with your hands and upper body to gently place head on the ground.

5. Straighten arms, lifting head off the floor.

6. Press all four corners of feet and hands into the ground, creating a graceful, flowing arc.

7. Let the head relax and neck lengthen toward the ground. Relax your face and jaw.

8. Draw Mother Earth's energy up through the hands, feet, and head.

9. Feel the unique openness yet strength this posture offers you.

10. The rainbow is present within you now. Feel each color radiate through.

Hold up to 15–30 seconds—about five big breaths through the nostrils only.

Benefits and Systems Being Treated, Challenged, and Healed:

• Builds self-confidence.

• Stimulates nervous system and endocrine system.

• Tones uterus and ovaries.

• Energizes body.

• Improves blood circulation.

• Increases body heat.

• Irrigates kidneys with fresh blood supply, assisting in elimination of toxins.

• Strengthens lungs and facilitates deeper breathing.

• Tones abdomen.

Precautions and Contraindications:

- Low back and knee muscles.

- Wrist limitations.

- Stroke, glaucoma, heart disease, or high blood pressure.

Modifications:

Place your hands on each side of your ears, fingers facing forward. Lift up onto your head but do not lift into full expression of posture.

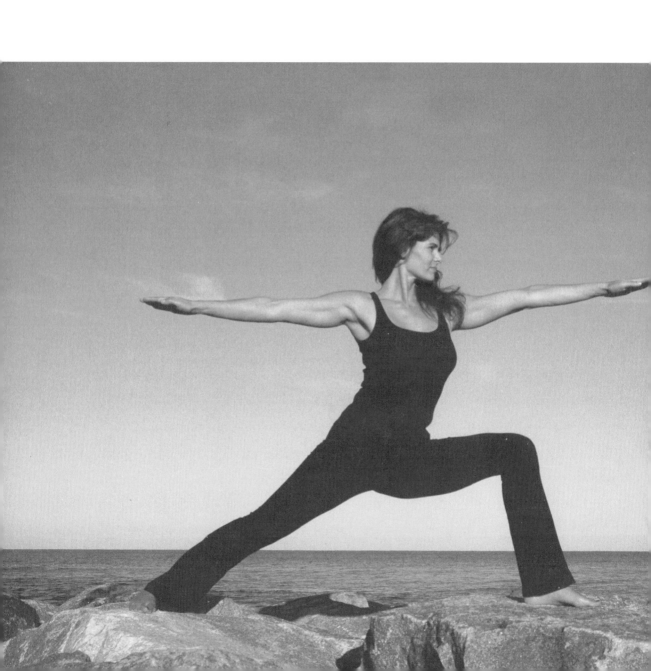

Chapter 5

THE PHYSICAL BODY

D o you know what you are doing, why you are doing it, and how it is affecting you? These are simple questions I always ask the women I meet at boot camp. Many do not know the answers, because they are just following what social norms and the fitness, medical, and beauty industry feed them. Ask yourself if you truly believe in what you are doing, or if you just do it because it is the easiest thing to do. You must be accountable for understanding your own body's intelligence before you can even think of having a strong and vibrant physical body.

The tools we discussed in the spiritual, mental, and emotional bodies have a synergistic effect that cumulates in the physical body. Our culture tries to work from the physical to the spiritual, while native cultures work from spiritual to the physical, knowing that their connection to Spirit is their power, and with power comes responsibility—to have a flexible mind, a strong heart, and physical stamina to move through life to be of service to Spirit. I cannot think of a more powerful, fit, and healthy model for living.

The spiritual, mental, and emotional bodies are subtle bodies, which means they are composed of unseen energy. The physical body is the densest body and is a concrete manifestation of our energy. As you think about your physical body, go back to the spiritual, emotional, and mental bodies and remember: *How I think is how I feel. How*

I feel is how I behave. And how I behave is what I create in my life—even physically. We must remember that our thoughts have that much power. If we are having an average of 50,000 thoughts a day and most are negative, then you know unhealthy manifestations will be the result.

It frequently happens that women come to me thinking that I will inspire them to get on track with a great physical workout, thinking that if they look good on the outside, they will feel good on the inside. I turn the tables on them: we start from the inside and work our way out. The truth of the matter is that their energy is stagnant; they are not able to move freely, because they stopped expressing themselves and started suppressing their own desires. They falsely think that losing weight will solve this problem, but they have not yet realized that they have lost themselves.

When you figure out where your life is off-track in all three of the previous bodies, losing weight will become that much easier, because you will lose the baggage that has taken up space in your system, which is showing up in your physical body. Weight is an aftereffect of energy not flowing and working at its true, healthiest potential. When the energy in the subtle bodies is stuck, the cells within our physical body do not vibrate at their highest frequency, which makes the blood flow less. On the physical level, blood carries oxygen, and oxygen burns fat in the simplest form.

On the emotional level, the feelings we suppress lead to more stress, which leads to making unhealthy food choices such as eating sugar, carbs, and caffeine to energize our bodies while we numb out our emotions. But all that sugar, high-carbohydrate food, and coffee overloads the nervous system and brain, which can create tension and insomnia headaches in the mental body, thus creating less oxygen flow. You also run the risk of completely turning off your senses and intuition—the body's intelligence that tells you when you are hungry and what your body needs. Spiritually, when your energy is stagnant, you lose the connection with your higher self, which intuitively knows what is good for you, whether it's healthy food, well-balanced relationships, appropriate geographic locations or certain surroundings, or rejuvenating activities.

One of the most common problems I see today is the "zoning out" that happens when people feel dissociated from their bodies. Zoning out is the state of removing yourself from your fundamental wants, desires, and needs and not fully inhabiting your own body. When this happens, you no longer know what is right or wrong for you; you just go through the motions of life and become a robot of accomplishment. It's true that some people get satisfaction when they check off the next item on their list of things to do. That joy can even drive them to set unrealistic goals to accomplish more and more, which can lead to stress of their own creation. Perhaps this joy is the only joy they feel in their life because of bad relationships, childhood, or marriage. This constant driving and striving keeps us from dealing with our fundamental issues and truly feeling joy, stillness, peace, and love. Sometimes we create in order to avoid feeling. Of course, I don't mean to say that creativity and accomplishment aren't healthy forms of self-expression. When this drive is unchecked and unbalanced, I think that the conquering of tasks and building of empires can unfortunately become less fulfilling than time spent alone or with loved ones.

As a culture, we have mastered wealth, but we haven't mastered health. When we choose to zone out or work on autopilot, Spirit cannot stay and do its healing work. Stress creates discomfort, and discomfort leads to zoning out. In medical terms, discomfort in the body creates dis-ease, and dis-ease manifests in illness.

Unfortunately, in many cases, we can become so disconnected from our physical body that pain is our only wake-up call—and often deep pain, at that. Pain is our body's way of urgently drawing us back to the present moment and to our physical body. A great example of this was when my uterus ruptured. I actually thought I had just pulled a muscle! I had worked out that day with weights, doing squats and lunges. There I was, a semiprofessional athlete, personal fitness trainer, and model who worked out every day, ate healthily, and did everything I needed to do to be fit—yet how was it that I did not feel my uterus rupture? How sick is that? I laugh about it now, but it was a painful realization. I was so far removed from my body that exercise was a way to force myself into an unrealistic model of being fit, beautiful, and powerful. As you can see, I know this deeply: in order to hèal, you must feel. When you feel, you inhabit your physical body.

Believe me, when you do the work that your pain calls you to, Spirit follows through with a great reward. It is the law of energy, of cause and effect. Healing yourself and improving your life is not rocket science. It's all about aligning your innate wisdom with the beautiful energy of the universe. This is when your burdens are lifted, and you realize that you are not alone. This incredible process creates flexibility, suppleness, and full range of motion in all aspects of our being.

Next time you are walking down the street or have a business meeting or dinner date, walk with your head high, reaching toward the sky, and connect to God consciousness.

Squeeze your shoulder blades; open your heart, connecting to Christ or love consciousness; and ground your feet firmly, as if you had roots growing deeply into the earth, connecting to Mother Earth consciousness. Doing this, you will discover your *hara*, or your core. This new awareness and attitude will glow from the inside out—and people will notice. I call it the goddess glow, showing that you are a radiant, beautiful, powerful being open to whatever the universe has to show and give you.

In scientific terms, we can explain the realignment of the physical body through Einstein's zero-point energy theory. Zero point is reached when a cell of the human body is working and vibrating at its full potential—when it has reached its ground state. An atom emits a glow of light. The radiant field, or the body of light, demonstrates the health of a cell, which resonates a frequency. This is why some people can quickly regain health and some cannot. Everything alive has a frequency that we can measure through our senses of touch, sight, sound, taste, and smell. It only makes sense, then, that the food we eat, the environment we live in, and the people we surround ourselves with can either feed and speed up our frequency or slow us down. We all know what fast food can do to us, compared to a fresh salad picked out of the garden. We also all know what it is like to be around an angry person compared to a joyful one. Which one attracts you, and which one repels you?

Our four bodies speak to one another by radiating frequencies that either support our health and growth or dampen it. When the spiritual, mental, and emotional bodies are healthy, the physical body manifests health and becomes more vibrant, too. Our smile, our eyes, our posture, and even our skin, which is the largest organ in the body and most sensitive to energy, sends off a positive, attractive frequency. This is part of the realignment process will naturally affect your relationships, too. A healthy, vibrant woman recognizes that all creatures are special and come from the same higher source, the light of God (or whatever you choose to call it). She does not judge people, places, or things as good or bad but as whether or not these things are of service or not of service to her. This is the power of self-love and understanding that love is life force. To live otherwise is to attract people who are unbalanced energetically, often called energy vampires because they "feed" off someone else's positive energy rather than generating their own. We need to attract people into our life who are energy generators, not energy feeders.

By removing toxins and stress in our lives, we give our energy permission to be free and to cleanse anything within us that does not serve us. This includes empty distractions such as television shows, commercials, the pressure to be fashionable and shop for the "right" things, and constantly checking our email and text messages, and spending too much time online. I don't mean to say that all of these things are "empty," of course—it's using them in such a way that they keep you from experiencing your true self and avoiding your own issues that's the problem. If you need constant stimulation from outside sources, how can you ever learn to truly stimulate yourself?

It requires discipline and commitment to create harmony and balance within, and this discipline requires you to stop, look, listen, and feel on a daily basis. We need to carve out time to retreat, to meditate, and to pray, to move our attention inward to gain insight and strength to move forward on our path. This action is a tune-up of our physical, mental, and emotional bodies, to bring us into alignment with our spiritual self. It is a tool to release toxins in the physical body, a practice to learn how to focus and concentrate on healthy thoughts for our mental body, an outlet to let go of worries and pent-up emotions that create stress in our emotional body, and nourishment for our spiritual growth and spiritual body.

When we take the time to create a space to purify and cleanse ourselves, we regain a sense of our center, our personal energy and power. This process will help you understand how to use your intuition, instincts, and senses as pathways to harnessing your body's natural wisdom, leading to a healthy physical body.

Goddess of the Physical Body
ARTEMIS/DIANA

The goddess of the physical body is Artemis, the goddess warrior also known as Diana in ancient Rome. Artemis is the goddess of selfhood, the Greek Olympian goddess of archery, daughter of Zeus, and sister of Apollo. Known as the goddess of the earth and childbirth, she influences health and grants health to others. She is the huntress who is one with the wilderness and wild animals, the protector of young girls. She is feminine in all aspects and was never conquered by love or marriage. Her sense of self and love for the divine are her main loves. She is also the oldest and most widely known and worshipped goddess across the globe, dating back to the New Testament.

Feared as much as loved by many, Artemis is true to herself and her purpose. She stands in her power and uses it to help others. She is a woman of truth, of purpose, and possesses a strong sense of self that keeps her on target and on her path.

Message from This Goddess[22]

I am who I am and know who I am. I know I can take care of myself under all circumstances, and I can let others care for me; I can choose. There is no authority higher than my own; my powers of discernment are finely honed. I am autonomous; I am free from the influence of others' opinions. I am able to separate that which needs separation so a clear decision can be reached. I think for myself. I set my sights and aim my bow, and my arrows always find their mark.

How This Goddess Works in Your Life

Feeling burnt out, "fried," and depleted? Afraid of being alone or not loved? Are you are a worrier or a warrior? Call on goddess Artemis, the goddess of self. She represents all aspects of the feminine goddess warrior within you. She is the huntress who shoots her arrows and reaches her goal.

Descriptors
FOR THIS GODDESS

Uninjured, healthy, vigorous, strong, healthy, focused, disciplined, compassionate, devoted, self-worthy

Have you forgotten or lost focus on what you desire, require, and deserve? Are you overloaded with chores and others' burdens? Have you fallen into the role of being codependent or settled into a relationship because you do not want to be alone? Let Artemis help you set yourself free. She will bring you back to your core. Allow her to help you focus on you. This is not an act of selfishness but of self-love. Realign yourself with Artemis's target to reach your dreams. She is the huntress of the forest and knows that love not only comes from humans but Mother Nature, so she is always connected to a source of power she can draw from. Artemis stands alone but does not fear her freedom, for she knows that her freedom means more to her than the love of a partner. She is never alone, for she has nature and her Amazon sisters. She does not fear individuality but rejoices in her freedom of self-love. To connect with her, take a hike through nature, rediscover your favorite animal, bathe in a river, learn how to identify trees, and run wild and free.

---

22   Used with permission from Amy Sophia Marashinsky's *The Goddess Oracle* (U.S. Games Systems, 2006).

What Is the Physical Body?

Like Artemis's powerful connection to nature, the physical body is ruled by the earth element, the body of Mother Nature. Unlike the other bodies, it is tangible and dimensional. The physical body is the easiest to understand because we can see it so clearly. At the same time, it is also the densest body and therefore harder to heal and keep in shape. It is the primary body through which we experience our many complaints.

The physical body is made up of atoms, DNA, and collective patterns that create matter such as our organs, glands, and systems that speak to each other to create our totality as a human being. Since our body is made up of the same elements as nature, the DNA of nature has the ability to heal us. That's why herbs, natural foods, and a healthy environment feed our body nutrients, oxygen, and vitality and create a strong immune system. Conscious living supports the systems of the body to function properly and to our maximum potential, which is the zero point. We must learn that our physical body operates like electricity, which feeds our electromagnetic field or our biofield, and in return runs through every cell of our organs, glands, and systems like electricity giving off a vibration, which creates a frequency.

How the Physical Body Operates Energetically

SCIENTIFIC THEORY: The body operates on electrical impulses.

ENERGY: Movement of electrical impulses with a positive or negative charge.

THE BRAIN: Sends a positive or negative message to the nervous system, and the body responds.

THE NERVOUS SYSTEM: The circuit system of action and reaction that sends a signal to all the major systems of the body (circulatory, respiratory, endocrine, skeletal, digestive, reproductive, etc.), entering deeper into each organ and gland of these systems.

THE HEART: The pumping action of our blood and energy determines how fast or slow our energy moves.

THE BLOOD: The essence of our being. The flow of our blood creates a current; this current creates a rhythm of our life force, which in turn creates vitality.

THE SKIN: The skin is the largest organ of the body and is the body's thermostat, the temperature control system. The feeling of sensations (hot, cold, numb, tingling, uncomfortable) are signals of what is going on within the body. These sensations tell us about how energy is moving or not moving in the body.

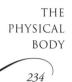

THE BREATH: The first thing to enter the body when we are born and the last to leave when we die. The quality of breathing is directly connected to the quality of life. The more naturally we can breathe and move, the more energized we become. As the body, mind, and spirit begin to function together, the physical body feels more alive and refreshed.

THE CHAKRAS: Wheels of light and energy. There are seven chakras that are energetically connected to the physical, emotional, mental, and spiritual bodies. These chakras are receptors of energy that take in and release energy from the environment and universe. Each chakra is connected to an organ, body part, and emotion. The chakras are different colors of the rainbow, with an individual vibration of sound, smell, sensation, and taste. The chakras determine how we act or react to the energy of our environment and therefore create our reality on the physical plane.

You can see how when our energies in the spiritual, mental, and emotional bodies are not in alignment, they can radically alter our physical reality.

Muscles of the Physical Body

Connective Tissue

The body as a whole—the organs, glands, systems, tissues, and cells (including the nucleus and the strands of genetic material, DNA)—are a continuous fabric: a matrix within a matrix. This matrix is connective tissue. K. J. Pienta and D. S. Coffey, at Johns Hopkins University School of Medicine, refer to it as a "tissue tensegrity-matrix system." The human body is a continuous network of tensional elements (ligaments, tendons, fascia, muscles, and cellular microfilaments). When a vibration is introduced to the body, it is quickly conducted throughout the entire system.

Connective tissue gives the body its overall shape and features and defines the form of each organ, tissue, and cell. All movements are generated and conducted within the connective tissue, which provides a physical, physiological, and energetic network for communication throughout the whole body. The nervous system is the most widely studied communication system in the living matrix, but it is by no means the only one.

This communication to the cells of the organs, glands, and systems creates a vibration, which gives off a frequency, which travels through the connective tissue, sending information.

The frequency changes every time a cell moves or alters its shape, an organ shifts its functional state, a muscle contracts, a gland secretes, or a nerve conducts an impulse. Transmission of vibratory signals through the connective tissue creates patterns relaying messages to and fro, alerting the connective tissue of the organs, glands, and system of the activities taking place.

Disease, disorder, and pain arise when the information does not flow, creating restriction and friction. Restrictions occur because infections, physical injury, and emotional trauma alter properties of the connective tissue's fabric.

The connective tissue retains a record, or memory, of our experiences, which is known as cellular memory. When the vibrations of our experiences pass through tissues, they are altered by the signatures of the stored information. Therefore, our consciousness and our choices are influenced by memories stored in soft tissues.

An important property of the connective tissue is it has an ability to regenerate, or to restore, itself. Massage therapy and other kinds of bodywork facilitate these processes.

DNA

Cells are the basic building blocks of all living things. The human body is composed of trillions of cells. They provide structure for the body, take in nutrients from food, convert those nutrients into energy, and carry out specialized functions. Cells also contain the body's hereditary material, called DNA, and can make copies of themselves.

Planet Earth's existence dates back to 4.5 billion years ago, when it was mostly made up of vapors and poisonous gases. Approximately 3.9 billion years ago, the earth's surface cooled, and DNA appeared first in bacteria form in rocks—the grandfathers, as the natives call them, because they were the first living beings on earth. Oxygen was poisonous to this bacteria and took on its form through the molecules of water. Through this shifting of DNA in nature, it created algae and creatures that lived both in water and on land, the snake being one of the first. The strands of DNA have manifested in physical form, bringing up the question for many mystics, anthropologists, scientists, shamans, and natives of what is the true symbolism of the mystery and magic of the snake, scientifically and spiritually. This question has been researched through time itself.

DNA is the matter of transformation, just like the mythical serpents. DNA made the air we breathe, nature, and the diversity of living beings, of which we are a part. In 4 billion years, it has multiplied itself into an incalculable number of species while remaining exactly the same. DNA is shaped like a long single and double serpent, or a wick of twisted flax. Just as we saw with the caduceus symbol, in which the two snakes are intertwined, the root of the word *twist* is two, twin double and wrapped around itself—the likeness of a rope or vine, the vine being the rod, the ladder that connects heaven and earth.

The ancient Egyptians, the Shipibo people of the Amazon jungle in Peru, and the Australian Aborigines have all used plants and herbs to open the doorway of the human mind, body, and spirit to tap into the DNA of the universe and receive information to heal diseases such as cancer and speak to the spirits. The shaman can see the patterns of DNA strands, their mutation, and where disease has manifested in the body. This vision can bring awareness to where the shaman needs to help the person and bring balance back to the DNA that has shifted. A common plant used by the Shipibo people is ayahuasca, which is a botanically and chemically complex hallucinogen with healing properties. Scientists have known for over a quarter of a century that molecules such as dimethyltryptamine and psilocybin from this plant resemble the neurotransmitter serotonin, and that serotonin increases DNA synthesis. DNA could transmit visual information through photons, which is visible light. This is another explanation of how some of us can see spirits and some cannot: our DNA gives off energy from our electromagnetic field through the vibration of our cells giving off a frequency. To shamans and in physics, this frequency can be seen or felt because of the receptors in the brain, just like when you go a psychic and they can read your aura and colors—they are reading the colors of your electromagnetic field. It is like fine-tuning a radio station to see colors, find spirits, and hear them speaking. Once we tune in to their frequency, we are able to see deeper than the physical.

This was true for me when I passed over to the other side in my near-death experience. I could see everything—how the universe worked, the simplicity of life and nature. How we are part of this huge element that is woven like a spider web, each strand connecting to galaxies. It was so simple, and the funny thing was I knew this to be true in every ounce of my being.

When I returned to my body, as I wrote about earlier, I could see things and feel things that I never did before—and still do. The DNA in my body was aware of the constricting patterns in my life—the people, the chemicals, and the environment was all too toxic for me and what I needed at the time. There was not enough oxygen for me to vibrate at the frequency of love I had experienced on the other side. I felt the walls were closing in, and my only savior was nature, where I could breathe and expand my body and my new consciousness. The DNA in my four bodies needed an oxygenated space to grow and evolve.

This is how I found nature to be my most powerful healer. This is what led me to work with the yoga masters, Native Americans, the Quero of the Andes in Peru, the Shipibo people of the Amazon, and the Australian Aborigines. What we must recognize and ask ourselves is: How could nature *not* be conscious if we are made up of the same DNA as nature? How can we grow and evolve if we do not have a connection to nature? How can we heal if we are not conscious of the resources that feed and heal us? How can we become conscious if we are not connected to the consciousness of the earth, where our DNA first came to life?

As we discussed in relation to the mental body, the more serotonin in the brain, the more intuitive we are. The more intuitive we are, the more we feel connected to our higher source. The more connected we are to our higher source, the more we feel at peace and act nonreactively. The more intuitive we are, the more we are able to tap into the consciousness of the earth and all its properties. As high as we go, we have to be able to go just as low, which then creates our bliss and reality in this world as we know it.

To put it all together: DNA creates oxygen, emits an electrical frequency of light, and creates the consciousness of a cell. Disease cannot live in an oxygenated, or conscious, area. By exercising, breathing properly, eating healthy food, and connecting to nature and its resources, such as herbs, we have everything we need to be healthy, happy, and abundant. This is so simple yet so complex for some. Isn't this what our nation is now trying to figure out as the human species evolves to what is already embodied in its DNA? This is why the natives believe we have to slow down in order to catch up.

Where there is oxygen, bacteria cannot live. Where there is no bacteria, disease cannot live. Where there is consciousness, there is love. Where there is love, there is life.

The Main Systems of the Body

By knowing how the body works and where our systems are, we can understand the mind-body connection, therefore opening us to the body's natural intelligence to heal. If you do not know your own body and how it works, you cannot heal or answer the critical questions of *what are you doing* and *how is it affecting you?*

SKELETAL

Bones make up 18 percent of our weight. The skeletal system is also made up of bone marrow, muscle, and soft tissue. We have about 600 muscles, making up 40 percent of our body weight. Connected to the root chakra.

MUSCULAR SOFT TISSUE

Muscles are attached to bones by tendons. Ligaments attach bone to bone, as in the spinal column, joints, and skull. The fascia is a connective tissue sheath that wraps around groups of muscles throughout the entire body. Connected to the root chakra.

NERVOUS

Nerves communicate with each other via electrical impulses that travel down the spinal cord, talking to each organ, gland, and system of the body, which are then connected to all the chakras. However, the fight-or-flight response is started in the adrenal glands when the brain perceives danger. It is driven by the root chakra and actualized within the solar plexus.

RESPIRATORY

Made up primarily of the lungs, which take in about a pint of air with relaxed breath (around fourteen each minute). The trachea, or windpipe, splits into two large tubes, the bronchi, one going into each lung. The entire structure is called the bronchial tree, consisting of alveoli, which constitute the bulk of the lung tissues. Located in the heart chakra.

CIRCULATORY/LYMPHATIC

Made up primarily of the heart, built of thick and tough muscle. The heart is the size of a fist and weighs less than a pound. The heart pumps blood through 60,000 miles of blood vessels. Mediated by red blood cells, blood's main function is carried out on a cellular level. White blood cells fight off foreign organisms and create white blood cells in bone marrow. The thymus gland is the center of immune dysfunction. The lymphatic system fluid carries waste away from cells.

Digestion and Elimination

The digestive system regenerates faster than any other system in the body. Even before the first bite, the smell and sight of food prepares the body to take in the meal or be repulsed by it. The mouth and tongue are activated by the secretion of saliva as enzymes are released for digestion during chewing and swallowing. The esophagus leads to the stomach and pushes food along. The walls of the stomach churn the food, mixing it with enzymes and hydrochloric acid strong enough to burn holes in carpet. The stomach protects itself with a layer of mucus. It takes two to three hours for food to travel through the stomach.

Reproductive

The female's reproductive organs are the vagina, uterus, fallopian tubes, and ovaries; eastern Indians call this the yoni, the nectar of life (which sounds much sweeter and more sensual than "vagina"). The female's reproductive system, unlike the male's, is located entirely in the pelvic region, the lower abdomen. The female reproductive system enables women to give birth, have sexual intercourse, and create eggs for fertilization. The gonads of the female produce eggs, and the male gonads produce sperm. The mother's egg and father's sperm pass along characteristics, called genes, to the next generation.

Endocrine

The endocrine system excretes chemicals and hormones directly into the bloodstream and consists of the pineal and pituitary glands, which are related to the third eye chakra and control the function of the thyroid gland (the throat chakra), which regulates metabolism. The parathyroid gland, also in the throat chakra, controls calcium and phosphorus balance in the blood. The thymus gland, located on the heart chakra, regulates the immune system.

The adrenal gland is connected to the solar plexus and is responsible for the fight-or-flight response, estrogen, progesterone, testosterone, and cortisol. The ovaries carry eggs and the prostate, sperm. The uterus holds the fertilized egg, and the testicles make sperm. They are connected to the root chakra.

Muscle Memory, Cellular Memory

"Cellular memory" is defined as the capacity of living tissue cells to memorize and recall characteristics of the body from which they originated. In the past, cellular memory was only thought to be stored in the nervous system, but biologists are realizing that all cells in the body have the capacity to store information in the cytoskeleton, referred to as the nervous system of the cell. Memories stored within any individual cell are accessed and communicated via the living matrix. The living matrix is best described as a web. Visualize how a spider weaves one thread together to create a web. The living matrix weaves together all creation; we are all one and connected.

Each cell of our being can store and process information like a computer. These memories stored in the cells can cause an action or reaction. What can trigger the action or reaction of a cell can be a pleasant or unpleasant response stimulating the fight-or-flight response, leading us to reaction or a calmness leading to action.

This is where most of our karma lies—in how we act or react to a situation. Imagine if you were brought up in a home that was verbally abusive, with arguing parents who tended to yell at each other, with never a calm moment. As a result, your nervous system and every ounce of your being would not be able to handle when someone yells or raises their voice. As an adult, you might end up attracting an argumentative partner who also screams and yells—and you are forced to shut down when it happens or fight back by screaming. The question is: Why did you choose this partner if you know that you could not handle it when you were a child?

The only reason the past can repeat itself is if we don't do the work of releasing our past trauma. When part of a negative experience has not been fully felt, without reaction or judgment, it remains stuck within us on a cellular level. As we work with the feelings and the sensations of these past traumas in a loving and supportive environment, we can embrace them in the present and experience and express our emotions in a healthy way to forgive ourselves and those who have hurt us. This process psychically and physiologically reprograms the nervous system to lose the reactive energy charge that causes us to overreact. When this charge becomes nonreactive and neutral, this part of life can be fully assimilated and integrated, bringing us back into alignment with our true divine self.

In the process of letting go of cellular memories, a lot of fear might arise, because the mind often does not allow what the heart wants to feel. The mind will make the pain seem 10,000 times worse than the pain actually is. The mind thinks having this fear will protect you. The fear reminds you to never allow it to happen again, but you continually repeat it because it is a pattern encoded and stored in your nervous system, cellular structure, systems, organs, and glands. Every time you hear, see, smell, touch, or taste something that reminds you of the situation, it triggers a reactive or active response that creates friction, tension, and dis-ease.

When we return as closely as we possibly can to the time when we were children and learn to listen to our body, we put ourselves back into alignment with its native and natural intelligence. Eat when you are hungry. Sleep or rest when you are tired. Breathe in nature and always play. But as we all know, returning to that childhood state also brings up the issues stored in our physical body. When did you overeat because you lacked emotional attention? When did you become angry because of the way you were treated? When did you lose your voice and self-esteem? These are all common causes of our weight issues, addictions, abuses of power, and of course illnesses and issues stored in our tissues.

Now we can understand how a belief system literally can carry that much weight in our bodies, creating a pattern of mental sanity or insanity, emotional havoc or health, and physical health or disease. Think about how, at every trip to the doctor's office, you are asked what illnesses and diseases run in your family. If a disease was in your past generations, you also have the possibility of that dormant part of your DNA rising to the surface. This is the power of DNA.

Your emotional history is no different from your physical history. Every disease has an emotional profile. How you treat yourself and your lifestyle is what determines whether or not the darker side of your emotional past will rear its ugly head.

It is now being proven that women with breast cancer have a certain profile, with many of these women showing codependent tendencies and giving way too much of themselves. With chronic fatigue, there is often a lack of boundaries. With MS, there is often held-in anger and tension, which numbs the nervous system. Every disease has a corresponding emotion and a story to tell. When we feel it and validate it, we can heal it. If we do not find the courage to do this work, we become a victim of our own emotions.

Cellular Memory and Healing the Generations

When I opened my own Pandora's box of emotions in therapy, I was ready to dig deep. Get ready by asking yourself some questions. How much do you really want to heal? How deep do you really want to dig for that truth—because in the process you will find things that surprise you. The ugly secrets come out, but they also set you free forever. You have the power to heal not only yourself, but the four generations before you and the four generations after you (this is a Native American and shamanic belief). When we heal, we shift consciousness, and this will change the form of our DNA, our cellular structure, to its core—thus setting our cells, heart, and spirit free.

I dug deep into my family tree to find out what types of emotional patterns are found in the lineage that I came from. Of course, no one wanted to talk all that much about the past, but I did it by asking about my roots, not the dysfunctions. After all, I did not want to offend anyone—I just wanted to know who I am from the core.

I found out that one of my aunts was a closet drinker. One of my uncles committed suicide. When I questioned my grandmother at age eighty-six about the abuse I experienced, she was very angry and defensive, and all but disowned me. She was my second mother and best friend. Everyone in my family was angry about me finding my truth, my voice—but it was not my job to convince them because they were, in some ways, part of the dysfunction. I felt alone, lost, and attacked, but I knew it was only fear, for my truth was a piece of the puzzle of their own lives as well. When it comes to families, the Pandora's box of emotions is passed down from generation to generation.

Months later, before my grandmother died, she cried to me about the sexual abuse that she and her five sisters had experienced. We cried together and healed our pain. It is never too late. Protecting someone else for fear of finding your own truth is betraying yourself and them in the long run. It is denial of our existence. This is the power of healing yourself and the generation behind you and in front of you. You have that much power.

I now have five nieces, growing goddesses who are learning how to be true to themselves and free from past burdens. They will never be abused; this disease has been healed. The mindset of my siblings and family has become more full of light, conscious, and aware. This consciousness not only healed myself, it has healed my whole family.

We must truly understand that as we evolve and expand into the light, we also expand into the darkness. Again, as high as we go, we have to be willing to go just as low. Once we master this concept, it becomes our reality. We no longer create separation, knowing that all energy is from the source of God—some energy just has a higher frequency and some has a lower frequency. But source is source. The darker energy, which I like to call lower frequencies, just forgot how to shine and work to its true potential, which is a part of each of us. We cannot cast judgment against anyone else when we also harbor all forms of energy within ourselves. This consciousness creates a powerful form of non-judgment. Once you have this power, you can choose what is healthy or not healthy for you. You have the choice to move into it or away from it.

The fear of releasing bottled-up pain stored in our body can be overwhelming. We fear the crying will never stop. We are stampeded by the sensations moving through our body—the sadness, rage, and even craziness surfaces, and you might feel like you are going to die. And the truth is, a part of you does—the part that is no longer of service to you. The mask that covered the beauty of your spirit and soul is lifted. This is the powerful rite of passage, the shaman's death, which gives us the ability to connect and feel the divine source within us and around us. I always say that what goes down with our emotions always has to come back up. Be prepared, for it will come out of you. It's an emotional, mental, spiritual, and physical detoxification process.

Examples of Cellular Memory

As I discussed earlier, my near-death experience happened on Christmas Eve, 1995. And every Christmas since then, my body would feel the operation again. I would feel the pain in my organs and glands moving around in my body and my uterus, which was taken out of my body in the operation. Because it had completely ruptured, the doctor took it out of my body to reconstruct it and stop the bleeding while the other doctors were setting up for the operation. Just imagine it. As a result, I would feel a recurring surge of heat and sensations move through my body like lightning bolts. It took me years to heal this, and now I rejoice in giving birth to new creations that move through me. Instead of feeling loss, I feel gratitude for all that I have given birth to—Boot Camp for Goddesses for adults and teens, Goddess Sacred Tours, Yoga Teacher Training, this book, and many others. Boot Camp is now thirteen years old. I like to say that she is in high school, able to take care of herself, feed herself, and is independent in many ways. I do not need to watch her so carefully. *Goddess to the Core* is her sister, and she was the hardest thing I have ever brought into this world. She was six years of labor but well worth it.

I think you get my point. I healed my wounds of not being able to have a child by giving birth to other creations. I now am a mother to many who lacked loving experiences of their own. I am the midwife who helps women give birth to what they desire, require, and deserve.

In your own life, you can celebrate loss rather than mourn it. Everyone has a loved one, either animal or human, who has passed to the other side. Every time the date comes up of when you lost them, your body will start to mourn—but rather than allowing this to overcome you, you can rejoice in the gift of their life. Do a ceremony to call them in and validate the joy you shared. Change your perception, and you will shift your pain to joy.

As another example, imagine how a practicing tennis player will serve a tennis ball 500 times a day to program the best release of the serve, where to place the ball, how to hold the ball, and where the body should be at all times. After a time, from repeating this exercise, the body memorizes the pattern through its own intelligence. The patterns become encoded in the connective tissue and nervous system. This is why practice is the key to success, whether it be physically in sports, emotionally by learning not to react, mentally by choosing positive thoughts, or spiritually by doing rituals to remind us of our divinity.

Flexibility

How far you can stretch? How healthy are your bones and muscles? Don't for one minute think that *flexibility* is a term used only for the physical body. Do you have a flexible mind? Are you open-minded? Can you be flexible with your emotions? Are you consistently living in the same frequency of emotions, or do you allow yourself to feel more? Can you be flexible with your belief systems and not judge others' spiritual beliefs? How flexible are you *really*?

Let's see how far you can stretch your mind and redefine flexibility.

When we activate and validate our suppressed feelings—our memories and thought patterns that are locked in the unconscious mind and body—we are bringing the unconscious to consciousness. When we feel, we are becoming conscious—consciousness equals feeling, and feeling equals self-love. The highest state of consciousness is the highest state of feeling pure, unconditional love and joy.

As your consciousness awakens and grows, the reactive patterns stored in your nervous system and tissues diffuse. The physical body not only releases but erases these patterns. The freedom is then seen in the flexibility of the mind, body, and spirit. You have full range of motion in all your bodies, can move easily, your life force is more alive, you have more vitality, and you become happier. Let me show why.

When doing exercise, especially yoga, you are not only stretching your muscles—you are also stretching the nerve endings, reprogramming the nervous system, and reprogramming the fight-or-flight response. Stretching creates flexible muscles, because you are relaxing the nervous system, allowing the emotions and memories stored in the connective tissue to surface and release toxins, physically and emotionally. This action not only allows our physical body to stretch but also our mind and emotions. How many times have you seen someone cry in a yoga class? My students often beg me to stop taking yoga poses deeper, for they know the deeper the stretch, the deeper the awareness, which releases their fears and ego. Why? Because the deeper the stretch, the more your resulting deep breathing will release tension and discomfort stored within. The breath opens the consciousness of the cells, muscles, organs, glands, and systems. This consciousness on the physical level brings on more blood, which carries cleansing oxygen to help you release the toxins stored in your muscle tissues.

The next time you are confronted with an uncomfortable situation, breathe, count to ten, and encourage flexibility in your body, mind, and emotions. This allows you to be active, not reactive, because you are aware of how to move either closer or further away from the situation without judgment. This practice gives you full range of motion. A true athlete recognizes that flexibility is about flow, not force. A true goddess warrior knows that her power comes from the balance and flexibility of being in tune with her emotions as well as her intelligence, and she is graceful yet fierce, strong yet supple in her ways.

Immune System

The immune system is made up of special cells, proteins, tissues, and organs. It is a sophisticated defense system that protects the body against disease by identifying and killing foreign cells such as viruses, parasites, and other invaders. The immune system distinguishes the unhealthy cells from the healthy cells and tissues in order to function properly, and creates white blood cells to help cleanse invaders from the bloodstream.

Disorders in the immune system can result in disease. Immunodeficiency can either be the result of a genetic disease, pharmaceuticals, or an infection such as AIDS. In contrast, autoimmune diseases result from a hyperactive immune system attacking normal tissues. The immune system is connected to the thymus gland and lymph nodes. The lymph nodes and glands support the white blood cell function. The thymus gland is located in front of the heart, behind the chest wall, and is the center of immune function. The thymus gland has a critical role in the development of a child's immune system before birth and for a time thereafter. Usually by the age of two, the thymus gland has reached its maximum size, and the immune system is fully functional.

When all four bodies are strong, our immune system is strong, and we can destroy invaders such as bacteria and viruses much more easily and kill mutated cells before they grow big enough to become cancer. The immune system is a key element to keep us healthy physically, to prevent infectious disease, internal diseases such as cancer, and autoimmune diseases like MS and lupus. Stress on any level affects the nervous system, which then affects the ability of the immune system to work effectively.

Body Intelligence

Intelligence is the ability to understand and profit from experience—by acquiring, storing, sorting, and applying knowledge. Other terms have been used to explain body intelligence, such as innate, natural, or holistic intelligence.

The body consists of much more than organs, glands, systems, flesh, and blood. It is the container of our emotions, our memories of everything we feel and have felt. Like a computer, the body has the intelligence to store our memories of every experience we have endured throughout life and the wisdom to heal itself. The body is the material part of the mind, and the mind is the invisible part of the body. Heal the body, heal the mind; heal the body, and the mind heals itself. The body's intelligence is measured by how well it heals disease or illness and the emotional trauma attached to it.

The Core

What makes up the core, and how does it work? The front of the energetic body is the emotional center, our "feeler"—how we take in information from our environment. The back of the body is our will center—how we put our energy out into the universe from the information received from our environment.

The core of our life force and vitality sits in the center of our belly. The navel area in both the front and back of our body is where all the nerve endings meet from all the glands, organs, and systems in our body. Eastern Indians call it the hara; oriental medicine calls it our Dan Tien, or the Ming Men, which is translated as the "gate of life" because it holds all of our potential for life and contains the initial spark of life that expands outward to give power to the organs, glands, systems, meridians/channels, and substances of the body. It is the root of our physical destiny, as well as the foundation of our mental and emotional lives.

To find your core, stand in an anatomical position: place your feet hip-width apart, your arms at your side, palms open, the crown of your head reaching up toward the sky, and squeeze your shoulder blades together to open your heart. Now breathe. Feel your breath moving up and down your body. Now move your body weight forward from the waist. What happened?

It usually takes about ten guesses before people figure this out. Women often say their knees hurt, their neck is tight, their back hurts, or they feel defensive. These all may be correct answers, but the main component that these answers miss is crucial. When you moved your body weight forward at the waist, you also *stopped breathing*.

Now bring your body back to the center, in the original anatomical position, and what happens? I often see confused faces as women try several times to feel out the answer. Then the answer comes: *I naturally took a deep breath*; *I can breathe*.

The message for this exercise is to fundamentally understand, feel, and experience your core. We often hear the words *find your core, ground yourself, find your center*, etc. We intellectually understand what these things mean, but do we take the time to actually explore how these concepts feel?

I believe that one of the biggest problems we have in our culture is not being present in our own body. When we are in our core, we are true to ourselves; we know who we are and what we stand for. We know where our energy begins and where our energy ends. We come from a place of nonjudgment and know that we are connected to all sources above and below us. We come from a place of self-love, which enables us to respect others and their paths. We no longer fall victim to others' wants and needs. We are observant and translucent in our energy, and know what to do and when to do it; we trust Spirit will guide our next move. There is no more guessing, just listening and following through.

This core power is where we must always remember to stand. This is one tool that every woman has taken home that has empowered them. When we are able to truly be present in our body, we feel energy. We intuitively know what someone might say or do before they do it just by watching their body language, trusting our intuition, and understanding how to use our energy through our own body language. In some cases, we have to come around to admitting that we are too sensitive after we realize that we take things too personally and absorb others' energies like a sponge. We must understand how to put up our filters and know what is ours and what is not ours. In order to do this, you need to be fully present in your physical body to sense the energy circulating through your feelings and senses. Women have a knack for this, but we cannot use this gift if we are not in our body.

For example, invariably someone you know will say something that hurts you. Instead of absorbing this negative energy or taking it on, ask yourself this: *Is this my shit or not my shit? Do I need to absorb someone else's insecurities, rude comments, or projections?*

Do you remember that scene from *The Matrix* in which Neo, the main character, is attacked by bullets whizzing around him in slow motion, and he dodges all of them? His feet are firmly planted on the ground; he is flexible in his core, bending in all directions and coming back with the force of self-love and the attitude and mindset that nothing can penetrate him. This is the visual you must have when bullets of negative energy fly around you. By this I mean projections (at home, at work, and those you inherit from friends and family members), unhealthy thoughts, unnecessary demands from your family, and someone else's negative energy. In your mind, say to yourself that "this is not mine" as you engage your core.

What might throw us out of our core power: people, food, environment, emotions? For example, if someone attacks you verbally, do your best not to respond emotionally and create more drama. Instead, remember the negativity is their own, keep your body language simple, and say, plainly, "How would you like me to respond to that?" By doing so, you dodge the bullet of negative energy. I know this is a hard lesson to learn—but it's wonderful when you do. I call this "the other side of power."

When we have mastered observing our emotions and mind in the moment without reaction, we have mastered how to be in our core. We have mastered how to come from a place of self-love and unconditional love for others. This is the foundation of a healthy and vibrant being claiming her space—not just taking up space.

A Healthy Physical Body

To tap into the physical body's resources, you must understand that finding balance within is necessary for growth and happiness as a human and a spiritual being. A healthy physical body knows that balance is the key to power internally and externally, and that

Qualities
OF A HEALTHY PHYSICAL BODY

Balanced, supple yet strong, flexible yet firm, energetic, strong immune system, stamina, self-generator of energy, vitality, strong presence, radiates beauty inside and out, full range of motion, rehabilitative, vibrant

awareness is only useful if it points toward action internally or externally.

The physical body is our temple; the home of our spirit, soul, and God. Our body is the vehicle: as they say, *as above, so below*. The physical body is always a manifestation of the state of the spirit.

How you react to any situation becomes a pattern of life stored in our cellular structure, the connective tissue. Prolonging pain and suffering encourages you to continue opposing the natural flow and harmony of life—your true nature. The job of your true nature is to know what to allow and what to keep out of your personal space. It knows the balance of giving and receiving and does not judge others' emotions but knows what is healthy or unhealthy. A healthy physical body knows overexerting the mind and body can cause adrenal fatigue, injuries, impaired performance, and physical distress. A healthy physical body knows how to balance effort and action with stillness and silence, action and reaction. It trusts your innate wisdom, the instinct within you that knows the right choices and moves, the best timing, and helps you release detrimental stress by setting boundaries.

Qualities of an Unhealthy Physical Body

A medical perspective from Jeff Migdow, M.D.

Imbalances in the physical body/earth element are the most common manifestations of four-body imbalance, including headaches, backaches, bowel problems, heart problems, diabetes, cancer, fatigue, and insomnia. According to the Western materialistic model, when the cells in the physical body break down due to internal conditions or injury, organ damage occurs and disease results. The cure is to take medication that reverses the cellular damage or suppresses the pain or have surgery to remove the damaged part.

The holistic perception is very different. In this ancient model, we are all made up of four bodies, and imbalance on any level can cause physical disease. Just as a blow to the head causes a headache, emotional stress, and mental anxiety, mental anxiety and stress can lead to pain in the head. In fact, in my twenty-five years of practice as a holistic medical doctor, I have found that over 50 percent of physical disease is directly related to imbalances on the emotional, mental, or spiritual levels.

When I first meet with a person, we spend almost an hour talking—and it's amazing how much information comes out that reveals deeper causes of their physical disease. The homeopathic laws of cure state that a person isn't healed until they are balanced on all levels. In ancient China, a person would first work on their spiritual connectedness, mental tension, and emotional upset to discover if a cure could be found before doing direct physical treatment—that is, the physical body is seen as the gross manifestation of the subtler bodies, and until the disease is rooted out of the deeper levels, a true cure cannot occur. Holistic physicians are aware of this fact, and I've often seen people treated via conventional medicine who have suffered from one disease to the next as the deeper cause still remained.

On the other hand, we all know that if we have a physical illness, it can affect all the other bodies. Thus, the tools of a healthy diet, exercise, and yoga or some other physical/spiritual practice are always important to keep our physical body as healthy as possible.

Qualities
OF AN UNHEALTHY
PHYSICAL BODY

Stagnant, no vitality, sick, codependent, reactive, suppressed, numb, victimhood

Disease of the Physical Body: A Case Study

About ten years ago, I saw a thirty-five-year-old woman suffering from depression, fatigue, dry skin, weight gain, headaches, joint pain, anxiety, and periods of deep despair. All her lab tests, including thyroid tests, were normal. She had been on antidepressants and sleeping pills, tried various diets, and been in therapy for over five years, and because nothing seemed to be helping, she had been forced to take a three-month leave of absence from her job prior to seeing me. When we talked, I could see she had no reason in her life to be depressed and wasn't really active enough to be so exhausted.

It was obvious, though, that she was depressed, tired, and in physical pain. Her symptoms were very much like low thyroid disease. I had seen many young women in the past who were undiagnosed with similar symptoms who have had a low body temperature and responded to thyroid treatment. Even though her tests had been normal, we decided to have her check her thyroid a different way—by her morning waking temperature.

She took her temperature in the morning under her arm for five days, with the average being around 96.8, below the normal temperature of 98–98.6. From these readings, I assumed she had a chronic sluggish thyroid and prescribed homeopathic medicine to stimulate her thyroid to work more effectively. Within three weeks, her headaches were gone, her energy and mood improved, she felt reconnected to life, and her temperature had risen to 97.6. At this point, she had the energy to begin to walk outside for thirty minutes four days a week, joined a gentle yoga class, and improved her diet. She cut down on red meat, pork, junk food, and cola and increased her intake of vegetables, organic grains, and herbal tea.

After two months of treatment, all of her symptoms were gone, her old vitality had returned, and her temp was now 98 on waking. We continued the treatment for six months. She continued to feel well and went on with her life from there. During one of her later sessions, she confided in me that she had had a miscarriage about one month prior to the beginning of her symptoms. Most likely, the radical hormonal change had affected her thyroid in some way, leading to the borderline low thyroid disease.

Hers was a classic case of how a physical problem can manifest on all levels, and if tests are normal, it becomes very confusing as to where the cause may be found. Fortunately, with the help of holistic thinking and physical tools, she returned to her normal life.

I've also seen hundreds of women suffering multilevel physical symptoms of menopause and PMS, both caused by hormonal changes that also affect the woman's emotional balance, mental clarity, and spiritual connection. With these women, I have found the use of certain herbs and remedies, diet changes to balance the hormones, and taking part in activities that open us up to deeper balance, such as chanting, dancing, and drumming, all help them find a deeper, clearer balance in their lives, enriching their experience and opening them up to their deeper feminine self through the heart and soul.

SELF-TEST TO DISCOVER THE CURRENT STATE OF YOUR PHYSICAL BODY

The following questionnaire is designed to enable you to find your strengths and weaknesses in each individual body and discover which body is the most developed and which needs the most work. It is also beneficial for strengthening self-awareness—the key in being able to objectively see yourself clearly and from there create more openness, strength, and balance in your life.

Take time for each question and answer in a way that feels truthful to you. If you have areas where you feel like you aren't being honest, know that these are the places in which you tend to fool yourself. Usually these are the areas that need the most work.

Give yourself 5 points for *always*, 4 for *often*, 3 for *sometimes*, 2 for *occasionally* and 1 for *never*. Then add up your totals for each body and the grand total. This will help you objectively see where you stand in this body. As you move through this book and take the tests for the other bodies, you'll be able to see where your imbalances lie. We suggest you redo each of these questionnaires every one to two months to check your progress and give you time to reflect.

Questions **Key**: always (5 points), often (4), sometimes (3), occasionally (2), never (1)	
1. I feel fit, energetic, and healthy in my body.	
2. My body feels flexible and youthful.	
3. My weight and muscle tone are good.	
4. I do vigorous exercise (jogging, fast walking, tennis, etc.) at least four times a week.	
5. I do some form of yoga and/or stretching exercises daily.	
6. I choose to walk rather than drive whenever I can.	
7. I eat healthy, natural, whole food without additives.	
8. I avoid stimulants such as nicotine, sugar, coffee, and caffeine.	

Tally your score by adding up the points that correspond to each of your answers and jot it down in a notebook or journal. Although 40 is a perfect score, where you fall on the scale today is not as important as seeing your scores improve over time, both numerically and in relation to your other bodies (you don't want one score to be off the charts with others far behind, for example). As you test all four bodies, you'll begin to see how you can bring more balance to your entire being. If, for example, you scored a 36 on your spiritual body fitness and later realize that your physical body fitness is only a 14, you can use that information to bring those numbers onto a more equal plane, perhaps by meditating less and working out more.

AN INSIDE-OUT WORKOUT
FOR THE PHYSICAL BODY

The following tools and exercises are practices to allow the physical body full range of motion to energize, revitalize, and regenerate every cell of our being to achieve balance and connect to the earth element. All eight muscles of the physical body connect you to your body's intelligence and core strength.

Healthy Eating Plan
THE ART OF EATING VS. DIETING

First, let's start with the word *diet;* it is has the word *die* in it. Diets do not work and will never work; the vibration of the word *diet* does not sound alive, and it feels like a punishment that we are not able to have things our body may need or crave. The way we should be eating is to *feed* us life, not suffocate and poison our mind, leading to unhealthy choices. Let's change our perception here and use any of the following terms instead: healthy eating, conscious eating, eating for a way of life. This resonates better with the mind and the body, plus it is forever while you are still here on earth. Diets seem to be fads that come and go; you may lose the weight, but the hard part of a diet is always keeping it off.

Our body has its own off and on switch that tells us what our body needs and craves. Follow a child for a day and see how their body is constantly talking to them. They go through spurts of eating a lot and then nothing. They try new foods introduced to them and then reject the ones they do not need based on how their taste buds respond. When this switch is broken, we have lost our ability to trust our body's intelligence on a whole other level, but this switch is our intuition at its best.

To turn this switch back on, you must tame the stimulants that affect the nervous system, such as white and wheat flour, white sugar, white potatoes, milk products, too much caffeine, and too much alcohol. All of these foods create mucus that numbs our senses and slows down our energy. Mucus carries bacteria, which affects the immune system—and we wonder why we have such diseases as ADD, obesity, food allergies, and addiction. It is this simple: we need to eat foods that clean our body, give us more energy, and are easily digested. If not, your body becomes a toxic dump, leading to disease. You can do all the exercise in the world, but if you do not have a healthy eating plan to go with it, you are defeating the purpose of exercising, so throw in the towel and save yourself the burn.

All holistic medical systems consider a healthy diet to be a prime cause for good physical health and an unhealthy diet a major reason for disease. The Chinese consider that over 50 percent of disease is diet related, and the ancient Ayurvedic medical system from India used healthy eating as a main therapy. We all have different bodies with different genetics and lifestyles, but there are certain rules for proper nutrition and eating that support our physical health, including:

- Avoiding overeating.

- Avoiding rich, overly sweet, fatty foods that weigh you down.

- Minimizing food such as red meat and pork and other fatty foods that are environmentally toxic.

- Decreasing stimulants such as coffee, black tea, and sugar, which overstimulate organs and glands and speed up cellular destruction.

The best way to find your body's best eating habits is to experiment with different types of foods and amounts until you feel the lightness, vitality, and clarity that should occur after eating, rather than the usual tiredness and lack of clarity.

Fasting Detachment

Giving our bodies a rest from digesting food and allowing the body to remain in silence and stillness is a wonderful gift. When we do, we are better able to listen to our body's neural signals and understand our attachment to food emotionally and objectively. We can measure our food and caloric intake based on what is going on in our life emotionally.

I know this was true for me in healing my eating disorders. Years ago, I used food as an escape, as a companion, and as protection. I gained weight because of my fear of intimacy; food was something I could use to numb myself out. When I first moved to Santa Fe, about a year after my near-death experience, I did not have enough money to buy enough food to eat. I would eat only vegetables and fruit, and I was tired, cranky, and irritable because I could not satisfy my deeper emotional cravings with food due to my circumstances and limited resources. I had to sit with my pain and learn why it was there, why I was hurting so bad. The whole experience forced me to examine my relationship with food and realize that I was approaching it as a sort of addiction. I did not respect food and its life force energy because I never had to go without it before. Once I removed myself from the mindless routine of eating for emotional fulfillment, I was able to dramatically change my relationship to what I ate. Trust me—you can retrain your seemingly ingrained compulsions when it comes to food. Push yourself to rise above it and see it from an objective viewpoint.

One fantastic way to achieve this new perspective on what you eat is to go through healthy periods of fasting. Fasting helps you create the muscle of detachment necessary to review your diet intelligently and also appreciate what you have. It clears the mind of unhealthy thoughts and regenerates the digestive system and all organs, glands, and systems. It is an internal tune-up that gives you clarity in your heart and mind, in return strengthening your immune system and connection to Spirit. You become more intuitive and aware of your body's natural and native intelligence. Your senses are heightened, and so is your love for life. You become more evolved and involved with the preparation of your food, your environment, and Spirit, all leading to gratitude and abundance for all that you have and had.

Today, I bless my food and express my gratitude for its abundant life force. Next time you sit down to eat, say a prayer of gratitude and feel how that food nourishes and sustains you. Food is a living source that is here to nourish, heal, and nurture you.

Exercise

Most of us no longer have to engage in hard physical labor in order to survive. While this has its obvious benefits, we have at the same time lost our connection to the earth and to our body. The majority of us no longer need to cut wood, hunt, work on a farm, take care of crops, or feed the animals to exist. We have entire industries to do this for us, which is both a blessing and a curse. We usually spend the majority of our days working in closed office buildings with machines rather than living creatures, and many of us work out at the gym, inside rather than outside. If possible, work out, hike, walk, and do yoga outside as much as possible.

Exercise is the universal key for achieving better health on all levels of our life. Like any other animal, our body is made to move. Giving ourselves the time and space to exercise at least thirty minutes a day has so many deep, lasting benefits. The exercise can be anything you want it to be: fast walking, jogging, cycling, working with weights, dancing—any physical activity sustained for thirty minutes that deepens our breathing, quickens our heart rate, and makes us sweat creates release and relief.

For those of you who aren't currently exercising, ease into a regular routine by doing twenty to thirty minutes four times a week. Build up over the course of a few months to regular daily exercise, and start to push your limits a little bit each time. We have to understand that there is no other option. Look at it this way: feel blessed that you don't have to chop wood for the fire and carry water from the pump to your home. Instead, celebrate the body and the freedom that you have. Also, treat exercise as a precious time-out for your spirit. What many of us don't realize is that we do not exercise properly or breathe properly, which puts more stress on the body. While exercising, we might watch TV, listen to loud music, zone out on the treadmill, or create a feeling of alienation by spending too much time at the gym with routines and machines. And when exercise is second nature, many people run the risk of beating up their bodies to gain muscle and release tension and stress. Sometimes, these types of approaches to exercise can create stress, because we get stuck on autopilot and forced into increasing adrenaline highs instead of feeling where our body is at with it all. Don't get me wrong, I love to burn and sweat at the gym with my workouts and power yoga, but I must also be willing to give my body the opposite force and energy—allowing flexibility, suppleness, and stillness. This creates balance and mindfulness, and I can more easily breathe into the movements with conscious effort.

Benefits:
- Stimulates blood circulation.
- Strengthens the heart and lungs.
- Releases toxins through perspiration.
- Weight loss and maintenance.
- Diminishes the high blood sugar of diabetes.
- Lowers cholesterol and high blood pressure.
- Releases physical tension.

- Creates feelings of emotional well-being, mental strength, and spiritual connection.

Spiritual physical activities such as yoga postures, qigong, tai chi, aikido, etc., done properly, use the physical body in a way that is connected to the spiritual body and the universal energy of prana/chi/ki. Through the body's movements, you not only revitalize your physical body but deepen your connection to spiritual energy. The key to these practices is to do them with an attitude of reverence for both the physical body and for your connection to the Creator/Gaea. If done this way, you unite your energetic and physical self and create harmony and union.

Benefits:
- Movement connected to Spirit leads to deep revitalization of all parts of the physical body.
- Stronger healing force.
- Feelings of physical vitality, emotional strength, and spiritual connection.

Massage

As we activate higher states of healing, our bodies will want to go unconscious. This unconsciousness can take the form of physical and mental numbness or of actually going to sleep. Before this happens, we must take charge and demand that we stay in the present. By embracing our unconscious patterns and staying committed to our love/feeling process, all suppressed feelings, memories, and thought patterns will come to the surface.

With the surfacing of these feelings in the therapeutic process often comes a sense of physical heat. This heat melts the holding patterns in both the physical and emotional bodies. There is a law of healing that states as tension goes through a block, it produces heat. This is the heat of unconditional love dissolving the blocks that hold it back.

Deep, cellular impressions in the body can be released and healed with the use of touch. Massage is one tool that can heal deeply by going into the unconscious part of ourselves to bring our consciousness forward. By tapping into the connective tissue, we can erase the memories of trauma and past hurt and pain.

After my yoga teacher training was complete, I knew I needed to go into deeper layers of my consciousness to heal. I entered a scholarship contest to go to massage school—and I won. I was not surprised, because I knew Spirit wanted me to go deeper, and there it was. I went to massage school not to actually be a therapist, but to heal my deep wounds of sexual abuse. I knew I had to face my deepest fears and my demons on a whole other level.

In my training, my biggest challenge would be to do this type of work with both women and men. Because of my past, when I was touched by a man, my body was programmed to respond sexually. The guilt, shame, and cellular memory of being abused was embedded in every ounce of my being. I would hide it by controlling men and leaving them before they left me, for fear of not being loved. The way to protect myself was to numb myself out with liquor. If I was numb and outside of my body, I did not have to feel or be present with my partner. I was just using them as they were using me. The necessity of loving and nurturing touch was replaced by sex. I did not know how to touch or be touched.

In massage school, lying on the table in a submissive position with a man above me brought up my fight-or-flight response and continually brought all my shit to the surface. Just as when I started yoga class, all I did was cry for another month. I felt like jumping out of my skin; every day, I forced myself in a loving way to walk through the fire because I would never get an experience like this again for deep healing. I worked with every man I could, and they were all very compassionate and understanding. This action from them was healing in itself.

Once in our morning yoga classes while I was in child's pose, one man pushed down on my tailbone to assist me. I could hear his breath and feel the weight of his body over mine, which just put me in a tailspin. All the memories of abuse came up, and every cell of my being hurt, which led me to cry, and the poor man did not know what to do. Fortunately, this time I was able to observe myself—I did not disassociate from my body but remained conscious and aware as I felt the unconscious parts of myself being healed. During my training, I released all the shame, guilt, and filth that was stored in my body from head to toe. Massage training has helped me help others with the power of touch and intention.

Music

Since the beginning of time, humans have used music as a way to release physical stress and open up emotionally. Find an instrument that you feel comfortable with, and learn how to play. Make music, and allow your body to become one with the instrument—and see how the physical body opens and releases deep tension. If you choose not to play an instrument, find soothing music to listen to in order to release deep stress. Create an intention to play or listen to music at least three times a day to deepen its effects.

Benefits:

- Opens up the body to new movements and sounds.

- Releases deep muscular tension when we relax into the music.

- Relaxes the breath and nerves.

- Increases the immune system's ability to fight disease due to relaxed nerves.

- Slows the heart and can reduce high blood pressure.

BREATHING FOR THE PHYSICAL BODY

Detox Purification

For centuries, as part of their spiritual practice, many Native Americans have used the sweat lodge and Europeans have used the sauna. The process of sweating, praying, breathing, and singing combined with purification challenges both the human body and spirit. Before going into the spiritual world, it is customary to get rid of heavy emotions, worries, fears, and fatigue so Spirit can come through. Becoming purified aligns our individual spirit with the spirit of life, the great mysteries of the universe, and the void from which all creation springs. Purification is a transformational tool that integrates the wounded parts of ourselves. It is a way to clean house spiritually, mentally, emotionally, and physically.

For better or worse, the Western model of purification is usually limited to experiences in churches, mosques, synagogues, or temples where people come together to rejoice in the beauty of God or a power higher than themselves. We go to these holy spaces to help us wash away sin, ask for forgiveness, strengthen the sick, be grateful for the baptism of newborn baby and the joining together of husband and wife, and to celebrate the life of a beloved family member or friend. These places of worship are also good to retreat to when feeling confused or just as a place to go to feel warmth in your heart. The objects in these places are meant to represent something pure and to bring us closer to God. The statues, music, water, candles, wine, bible, priest, rabbi, minister, nun, etc., along with the intention of the people gathering in one place, is intended to purify our soul, spirit, minds, hearts, and bodies, both as a spiritual being and a human being.

In this way, most of us are taught to believe that God is something outside of us. We have been set up to believe that we cannot be completely whole until we have communed with the Almighty. In the Western world, this is when we are purified.

Remember that there are other forms of purification that a lot of us take for granted. When women have morning sickness, it is a natural way the body rids itself of toxins, so her body can be clean and pure for life to pass through her. When women have their monthly cycles of the moon, it is another way our bodies purify. The uterus sheds a sheath and unnecessary eggs to balance our hormones and cleanse our womb and our emotions. This purification and cleansing process is a special time when women are more intuitive, and it is also a time of reflecting, just like the moon. Our dreams are more intense, and our sixth sense is more sensitive, because our body internally understands that we are connected to something higher than ourselves. As women, we have the unbelievable ability to birth life, an experience that connects us to our higher self, God, and the god within us.

We use different techniques such as Lamaze breathwork to purify and cleanse our mind, to ease the tension of the muscles, to stay centered mentally and emotionally, and to take the focus off the pain. Most women have experienced all of these things I mention above. They are miracles and moments of self-awareness, enlightenment, and purification of our minds, bodies, and emotions. This is a natural act and a reflection of nature.

Purification from a Native Healer Point of View

Purification in the native language is a spiritual, mental, emotional, and physical tune-up, just like tuning the strings of a musical instrument and the practice it takes to attain its harmony. Purification is an ancient practice that has helped people connect to their spiritual paths. It is a detoxifying process that clears negative energies, which create imbalances in our system. Through the practice of purification, you can cleanse and bring balance to your mind, emotions, environment, and personal space (energy field/aura).

Purification ceremonies re-create time and space in a non-Western way to alter our ability to see and perceive things differently and to connect to unseen forces and spirits for guidance. These ceremonies are a time and place for prayer, to be still and silent, listen, ask for guidance, and receive answers—to surrender and let go of expectations and be grateful for who we are and the gifts we have received on our life's journey. Purification is a ritual, a symbolic act repeated to help people with their daily stresses and mistakes through the ups and downs of life. It is like riding a wave. Are you ready to reach the top of the wave? And what kind of wave? The wave represents a stage of some spiritual quest or level of energy. In the context of our spiritual quest, purification is reaching a stage of spiritual alignment. When we reach this stage, the individual spirit starts to manifest itself through our personality. We then start to walk, reflecting the colors of our own soul.

To attain this tune-up, it is necessary to do the following steps:

Step 1: Healing

Receive healing on all levels: spiritual, mental, emotional, and physical.

Step 2: Wisdom

Educate yourself with the wisdom of the native language of the path you wish to walk on, whether it be the Native American path, the yogic path, or the shaman path. This is the most challenging work—to experience and find the synchronicity with our spiritual quest and our life's actual journey.

Step 3: Quest

Start an individual quest into the spiritual world to receive your special spiritual gifts. These spiritual gifts are direct experiences that motivate us to reach our life's potential and purpose. These experiences nurture and strengthen our soul.

Step 4: Execution

To execute is to walk with our words, to "walk our talk," to make our dreams come true, and to share our wisdom. To learn, work, and share is what feeds the human spirit and soul. Once we have reached this stage, we are ready to surf the top of the wave. In other words, we don't need a formal purification ritual to go into the spiritual world, because we are an individual spirit in its human manifestation. When we have come to this place, we have found peace within and no more stress, heavy emotions, or crazy mistakes.

Connection to Earth

Everything is one, and we are all connected—so why do we feel a sense of separation in our lives? It's terribly ironic to feel separated from God, Mother Nature, and each other—the very sources that created us and sustain us.

What have we created in human society that has given back as much as we have taken? We can invent new ideas and machinery and tap into creative minds to solve problems, but we created these problems to begin with. Everything we have accomplished as humans uses the resources of Mother Nature to produce more money and come up with new inventions. And even though we have created the wonder and power of medicine to save lives, surgery to extend life, and massive vehicles to travel into space, time and again we have used God's creation, Mother Nature, and her resources to invent them. It is clear that we have not created anything as pure and whole as what was originally provided and created for us.

We cannot physically replace what we have taken. All we can do is give back our time, respect, prayers, and sweat. We can plant a seed, but we can't make one. In the planting, we show our respect, honor, intention, and love—but there is nothing tangible we can give back. It is not in the planting of the seed—not the digging of the hole and the placing of the seed in the ground—it is the action and the intention. This is what we can give back for what we have taken and how we can restore balance to creation.

Mother Nature is our biggest teacher. She is the creation of God and the true meaning of power. The great Mother Earth provides our life force, produces our physical stamina, and feeds all four of our bodies to stay alive. The sun that gives us light and the moon that reflects mystery and the void; the trees that give us fresh air to breathe; the fruits and vegetables that feed our body; the vitamins, minerals, and animals that provide food to fill our bellies—these gifts provide beautiful aromas, colors, tastes, and sounds for our senses. Her resources have provided the material abundance that our world has lived off of. Nature is a reflection of our being, a pure and natural source of energy. We are all just a living organism that holds a frequency that vibrates and gives off energy. But as a civilization, we have chosen to live unnaturally—and we are now truly seeing and feeling the damage we have created.

To find balance and come into harmony with Nature and life, we must learn to give thanks and be grateful for what we have. In doing so, we will weave in and out of the spiritual and physical to create balance in everything we do.

Exercises to Connect to Mother Earth
ACCESSING MOTHER EARTH'S ENERGY

1. Go outside.

2. Close your eyes.

3. Breathe in and out of your nostrils only.

4. Stand up. Come into alignment, with your head facing up toward the sky. Squeeze your shoulder blades, and open your heart. Plant your feet firmly into the ground, hip-width apart.

5. Feel the roots growing under your feet, connecting to the core of the earth.

6. Visualize an umbilical cord coming from your belly button and connecting to the core of the earth. There is no right or wrong way to do this; allow your intuition to guide you. Feel this connection deeply. Remember: the earth is your true mother, who provides, protects, sustains, and holds you in her arms.

7. You also can do this exercise sitting. Sitting under a tree, repeat step 4 with your tailbone pressing into the ground. Feel your roots extend from your tailbone, connecting to the core of the earth.

The core of the earth and the core of the human belly are made up of the element of fire. Through our core, we digest, integrate, and assimilate our food, our toxins, our emotions, and our energy. Our core is a wide-ranging clearinghouse and filter. With Mother Earth, when volcanoes erupt and earthquakes shake the foundation, she is detoxifying and expressing her emotions. Similarly, when we have problems with ulcers, digestion, and with our elimination, we are backed up and filled with too many toxins.

It may sound funny, but it isn't; natives know this to be true. Every course I teach, this is one exercise that women love and continue doing. This is one way to truly understand how deep a connection you can have with the earth. We must remember that as high as we can go up to the heavens, we must be able to go just as low into the earth to heal and come into our power, which now leads us to the next exercise.

Gaea/Mother Earth
THE CORE OF OUR EXISTENCE

This exercise reminds us to be present in our bodies, to stay grounded and connected to our core, to feel and connect with our environment and be grateful for its presence, and to feel oneness with the earth and her resources.

1. Lie facedown on the ground.

2. Lift your shirt up and connect your naked belly button to the warm yet cool earth.

3. Place your forehead (your third eye, right between your eyebrows) to the earth.

4. Smell the grass, feel the ground, and breathe in and out of your nostrils only.

Do this for at least five minutes or longer. You may be there for a while; it becomes addictive.

Your heart rate will start to slow down; with each breath, your body relaxes and starts to sink deeper into the ground, and the chatter in your mind is quieted. The earth is filled with minerals, and our body resonates with these minerals. When your heart rate slows down, you may even hear and feel the heartbeat of the earth. You will sense a vibration.

While you are doing this exercise, imagine the sensations of the earth with all of your senses. What would Mother Earth smell, taste, look, sound, and feel like? In your mind's eye (your third eye, between your eyebrows), visualize the color of honey—it is amber gold, the color of abundance and royalty. Real gold has healing properties. Now the texture: think of honey, sticky and gooey and full of nutrients. It is vital, sweet, changes color in the sunlight, and fundamentally fluid and sexy by nature. It is the nectar of the earth that attracts bees and fuels pollination. Pull up this energy from your belly button and breathe into your belly with five big belly breaths. Allow the nectar of Mother Earth to fill you with nutrients and vitality.

After practicing this exercise, you will naturally enhance your feminine essence, your own nectar. Like bees drawn to honey, you will have the goddess glow and will be irresistible. A woman who can go inside, be truly down to earth and natural, and feel completely comfortable and present in her body is very powerful and sexy. Watch the results.

Benefits:
- Detoxifies the physical and energetic bodies.
- Fills your body with vitality.
- Creates balance and harmony in the nervous system.
- Lowers blood pressure.
- Resonates with your energetic field, raising your frequency.
- Cleans your auric field.
- The skin soaks up minerals from the ground. Lying on the ground is detoxifying and helps us move back into harmony with nature, which brings our energetic field (also known as electromagnetic, or biofield) back into alignment and radiating a high resonance.

GODDESS STORY

As the master instructor of a martial arts academy, I am always looking for ways my students can use their leadership skills while getting involved with local charities and community events. Such an opportunity presented itself last year. We participated in the Relay for Life, the signature fundraiser for the American Cancer Society. We held various fundraisers for several months and participated in the twenty-four-hour celebratory event. The first year was extremely busy and stressful for me. I had tons to do and coordinate, and quite frankly, I was cranky, and it seemed that nothing ran smoothly. The event was a huge success and we were the number-one fundraising team, but my stress level was at an all-time high.

The second year was looming in front of me, and I had less time than ever to plan and coordinate everyone and all their activities. I was our team's captain as well as one of the chairpersons on the overall planning commit-tee. Surely, I had bitten off much more than I could chew! But having just spent two weeks at Goddess Yoga Teacher Training, I was eager to try some of the new techniques I had learned from Sierra Bender. I was searching for ways to incorporate all the yoga postures and hoped to spread my newfound knowledge.

As the day began, people were approaching me from all angles with questions, demands, and complaints. I felt my stress level rising, and I did what seemed to come so naturally: I lay down on the earth and allowed all the stress to just roll off my body. After a few minutes, I got up and carried on without any anxiety or stress. A little later, when my team got together to practice for our huge performance, their stress was palpable. So I immediately lay down on the grass and closed my eyes. They asked what I was doing. I replied yoga and suggested that they join me.

We all lay down on the earth, basking in the sun, as I softly suggested that they allow their bodies to sink into the earth, to let the ground hold them, and to allow all their worries to just melt off their bodies into the ground. A few minutes later, we began our practice with great, helpful attitudes. After this experience, anytime someone felt the slightest bit of stress, they came to me and asked to do yoga—which meant that we lay together on the grass. If they had a question or needed my opinion, they would come and we would have our discussion while lying on the grass. It became quite the thing to do.

Our performance was spectacular. In fact, I'm not sure who enjoyed it more, the crowd or us. Unlike the previous year, everyone was in great spirits, and the entire time was spent in a joyous, cooperative mood, interrupted with periodic earth hugs. (We even won several awards, including second place fundraising team, best campsite, and best youth participant.) After the event, when we were all tired and hungry, instead of rushing off to the nearest restaurant and then home to a hot shower and bed, we decided to join together for one last bit of "yoga." We all lay on the ground, giving thanks for the beautiful day and the wonderful feeling of a job well done. I felt such a strong connection to the earth and to my students; I can't recall ever having such a peaceful feeling. I knowing that this could have been the day from hell, and instead it became a true testimony to how feeling truly connected can make all the difference in the world!

I think it's worth mentioning that when I say students, I do not mean children. Those who joined in the grass "earth hugging" were all teenagers and adults. Children will often join in on things like this naturally, with not a thought as to how they might look to others. But when you have a group of teens and adults who are willing participants, well, it just proves that the technique works so well that nobody gave a second thought to joining us.— *Raea G. Pereira*

Goddess Story

I was introduced to the experience of Boot Camp for Goddesses by a friend. I thought it was exactly what I had been waiting for. My next thought was how I could justify the cost to my family and myself. I filed the thought and kept an eye on the registration date.

Four months prior to boot camp, I was approached by my father and offered $1,000, saying he had had a good year and wanted to give a little something to each of his children. I knew at that moment what I was going to do with this gift, so I registered and paid.

In the meantime, a long-awaited surgery was scheduled by my surgeon for five weeks prior to boot camp. I thought it would only take a couple of weeks to recover, then I'd be back on my feet as usual; then a kidney infection set me back, and my sacrum/hips locked up.

While driving to boot camp, I realized what a spiritual hit I took with surgery. I got to the intersection to turn to get to the site and got turned around so many times that I cried and wanted to go back to the security of my home, which I had been limited to for the past five weeks. I got to the site and faced another disorienting episode with finding my cabin and even unlocking the door. Ego and "willing it to happen" really get in the way with intuition and spirit work!

Each day at boot camp began with a silent 2.5-mile hike. I listened to my body and took it easy, and after about a quarter mile I took the shortcut back to my room to rest. The next day, I was delayed from the group and got lost, but I found the labyrinth, so justified to myself that this was where I needed to be. The following day, I passed up the hike and rested/walked the grounds, angry with myself that I could not keep up. You see, I'm used to keeping right behind the "lead dog," even if I had to struggle and ignore the pain or discomfort, I could always shut it off.

Well, the last day of the silent hike, I carried within me a sense of self-doubt, disappointment, failure, and defeat (when it came to this physical challenge). So we all started off as usual, and I vowed today to at least keep to the middle of the group. As each person passed me, I counted my position, then began to drop back due to a pulling pain in my right pelvic area. As I grabbed my skin there and pulled back at the pain, I had already been asking the universe (God) why am I here, what is my truth, and then I heard the voice of an oak tree. I initially looked up, thinking it was possibly an animal (like chatter from a raccoon, but higher pitched). I saw nothing but the tree, and I thanked it for being. As I continued on, soon after, another tree, a juniper, made the same sound. I stopped and asked, "Is this your voice? Then what do you want me to know?" At that time, I realized where trees' voices are: at the top of the trunk, where the branches begin. I also looked up the path and saw the last person disappear. I tried to hurry on but could not, due to the pulling pain. An immense, overwhelming flood of emotion overcame me, and I said out loud (which made it real), "I'm the last one, *I hate being left behind*, I was *always* being left behind!" It was not about being last. I stood bent over, as if the wind were knocked out of me, and began crying uncontrollably as these long-forgotten, repressed memories and visions returned of being around six to ten years old and being deliberately left behind or forgotten by my mom (my dad never knew or she lied to him to cover).

As I got older and tried to stand up to her, the hidden abuse and name-calling started. She would decide if she didn't like the way I looked that day, or if I disputed her, that I was a dog and would lock me out back all day, sometimes into the night until just before my dad got home. I learned to jump fences and had the immediate neighbors to go to (who did not tell on me or treat me like I was a heathen). One in particular was a young couple who had a baby girl; when I would knock on the door, the mother, Paula, would ask if I was OK, and I would tell her, "Today, I'm a dog." She would let me in and made me feel smart, reliable, important. She actually trusted me to help her take care of the baby, and soon I had my first baby-sitting job, and she got me many others.

When I was a preteen, Mom would tell me that I was invisible to her, and she could go days without speaking to me and could look right through me. Sometimes, I would be sent to my room even through meals, and when she would say I could come out, she would add, "Oh, are you hungry? Sorry, no food left for you"—and my siblings were not allowed to share with me.

The very hardships that we are challenged with in our lives can be our gifts if we let them, and mine has been about forgiveness and trust. Not only about others but mostly about whether I could forgive and trust in myself. Imagine my immense fear when I became a mother of two daughters myself. I promised each one at birth that the cycle will stop and a new one would begin with them. And that meant I had to forgive my mother—literally release her pain to the universe, because it was much larger than me and her.

That day (at boot camp) in the sharing circle, I wasn't sure how the women would take my experience on the hike or my story and I wanted, at least, to provide a lesson to come out of it. I encouraged each woman to notice a young woman, a girl—whether their own child, their niece, neighbor, or friend's daughter—and even if they seemed unruly, regardless of the reason, to try and advocate for them. Even if it's a simple act of trust in them or offering praise of something, *anything* positive in them. I took my neighbor Paula's simple and quiet encouragement, and it acted as my candlelight of hope in the furthest, darkest place. To her, I was someone important enough to be listened to and trusted. I named my first daughter's middle name after Paula's first daughter.

Later that evening, I was honored to share my space (my cabin) with the medicine man/shaman (who came to help with the labyrinth) and his family, as they needed a place to clean up from their travels, and I learned that the boot camp goddesses were all to help celebrate his daughter's first moon! What a beginning!

Sierra, this is my first time putting this in writing. It makes it real again. I believe you that it might help other women know their truth. It was more challenging than I initially thought.

Thank you with all my heart.

—*Elaine R. (BaBa Yaga Wild Woman)*

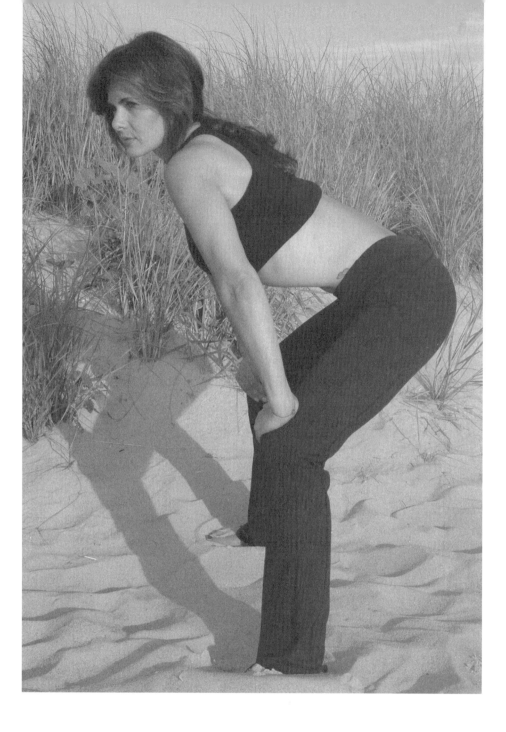

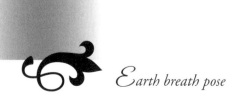 *Earth breath pose*

Earth Breath/The Stomach Pump
Sanskrit name: Agni Sara

The earth breath is the element of earth and nature. It is the breath of grounding and cleansing. All the major organs, glands, and nerve endings meet at the belly, which sits in the core of our body. The earth breath's pumping action lifts the abdominal muscles, therefore massaging all the internal organs and glands, feeding them fresh oxygen and blood flow.

1. Start in a standing position.

2. Inhale, place your arms over your head, and as you exhale using the ha breath (see page 204), pull the universal energy from above to your belly.

3. Come into a squat position, hands on knees, and relax your neck and head.

4. Hold the breath out, pull your abdomen in and up, and pump your belly button into your spine twenty times.

Goal: Four sets of twenty.

Benefits:

- Strengthens abdominal muscles.

- Stimulates the internal organs.

- Improves digestion and circulation.

- Rids the body of toxins, tension, pent-up emotions, and stale air as you exhale.

- Relieves constipation and irritable bowel syndrome.

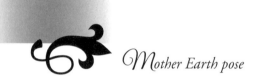 *Mother Earth pose*

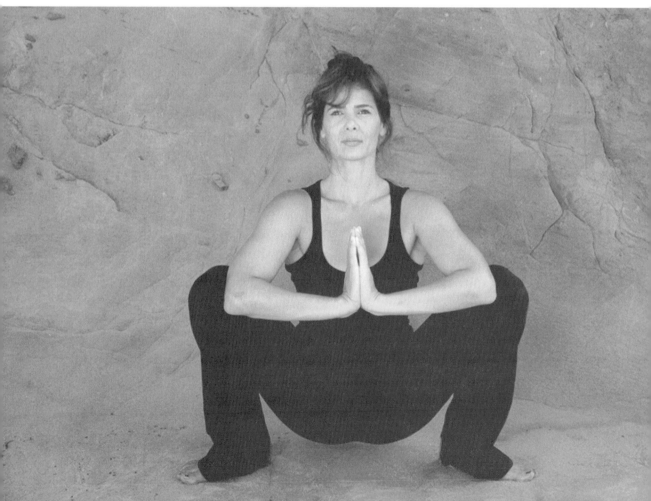

YOGA POSES FOR THE PHYSICAL BODY

Yoga is the science and practice of self: self-awareness, self-acceptance, and self-love. Each posture will reflect your weaknesses and strengths. Are you able to go into pain or do you run from pain? Breathe, have patience, and know that yoga is not about being flexible but being in the present moment so that you can stop, look, listen, and feel what is going on within. It is about intention, not perfection. The physical body will always benefit from what you do internally first and work its way out to the external.

Mother Earth/Life

Mother Earth gives birth to all creation. Her power is love, which creates rhythm and harmony in all of life. Her arms are always open to receive her children. Nature is a reflection of her beauty as well as the beauty within.

How do you reflect nature, and how does nature reflect you? What emotions are you harboring in your hips that block your flow and do not serve you? Are you flexible and supple yet strong? Spend time with Mother Earth; she will absorb your pain, agony, or despair and contribute to your happiness and health. Are you ready to love yourself as much as she nurtures herself?

Entry and Holding Posture

1. Come into a squat position, with feet flat on the floor. If you are having a hard time getting your feet flat, roll up the edge of a yoga mat or blanket and place under your feet for balance.

2. Place your hands in prayer in front of your heart and press your elbows into the inside of your thighs and knees to open the pelvis.

3. Press the crown of your head up towards the sky, drop your tailbone down towards the earth, and press all four corners of your feet into the earth.

4. Breathe in and out of your nostrils only, filling your heart, belly, and pelvic floor, your yoni, with breath.

5. Feel the expansion and tension we hold in the hips and pelvis.

6. Release the tension by coming into fire breath (see page 85); feel your body sit, sink, and melt into the earth. Remember, women gave birth in this position.

Benefits and Systems Being Treated, Challenged, and Healed:
- Strengthens core muscles of the pelvic floor and yoni.
- Strengthens the immune system.
- Stimulates the ovaries, sending in fresh blood flow.
- Enhances digestion and elimination.
- Strengthens circulatory system.
- Great for varicose veins.
- Strengthens the thighs and buttocks.
- Opens and flows your energy for orgasm.
- Grounds and connects you to earth energy.

Precautions and Contraindications:
- Bad knees: use care on the way in and out of pose.
- Hysterectomy (one month prior) and after any surgeries in the pelvic area.

Goddess/Empowerment
SANSKRIT NAME: UTKATA KONASANA

Goddess honors the your natural birthright to stand tall and claim your space. This posture reveals the goddess traits of mystery, magic, vitality, and beauty that live within the essence of your soul. The goddess offers the power to change. With her feet rooted to the ground, she stands firm, yet is flexible. As she stands in her true essence, her heart is open to receive, yet grounded to protect herself from what she will or will not allow in her space.

Are you ready to claim your birthright? Can you open to the power of the goddess, igniting courage to stand in your true authentic self? Do you stand in your own power, claiming your birthright?

Entry and Holding Posture

1. Begin standing with your feet together and your arms held outward, parallel to the ground, at shoulder height.

2. Using the ha breath, come into a wide standing position with your legs and feet turned out at a 45-degree angle and your arms still at shoulder height.

3. Bend your knees and allow your pelvis to descend directly downward without arching the lower back. Pull up on the pelvic floor by drawing the lower abdomen back toward your spine so you create a strong, stable core.

4. Press all four corners of your feet evenly into the earth. Move your knees toward a position centered over the ankles.

5. Bend your elbows at a 90-degree angle and point your forearms, with hands straight up and fingers spread wide, palms facing forward. Pressing into your feet, keeping a stable core, draw your body down as you open your thighs further.

6. Lift your rib cage, evenly creating space across your chest and back. Allow your shoulders to spiral gently backward and your shoulder blades to move down the back, opening the heart.

7. Lengthen up through the crown of your head, with your chin parallel to the earth and your eyes gazing forward. Find the center of the pose just below the navel, and allow your energy to radiate out, providing energetic support.

8. Come down into the pose further.

9. Using the power from your core, repeat the goddess mantra: "*I am a twenty-first century goddess. I am feminine. I am sensual. I am sexual. I am powerful. Don't ever mistake my kindness for weakness, and don't ever take me for granted. Ha!*"

10. Come into your fire breath (see page 85): for twenty breaths, breathe into your yoni, your female organs, and feel the fire in your belly.

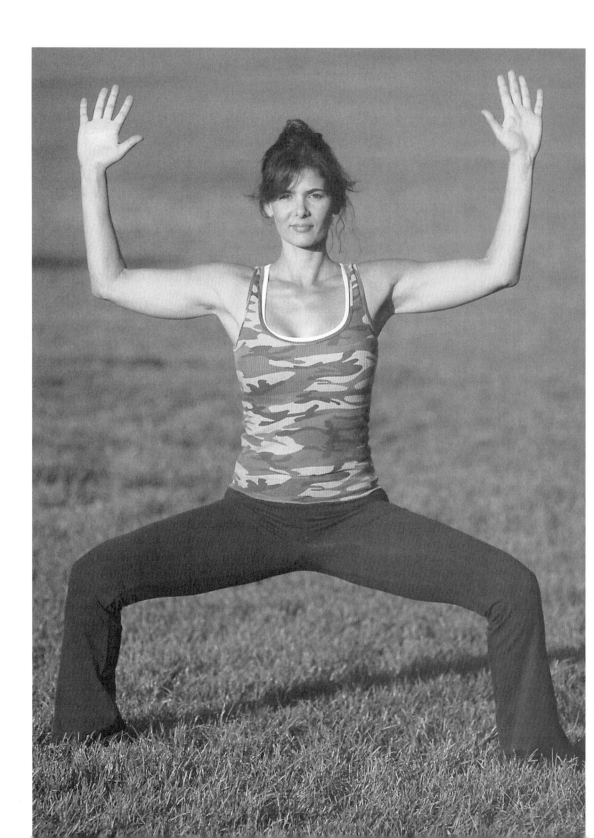

11. As you release from the squat position, bring your hands in prayer and feel the power of your own presence—a goddess to the core.

Hold up to sixty seconds—about ten big breaths through the nostrils only. Repeat two to three times.

Benefits and Systems Being Treated, Challenged, and Healed:

- Builds personal power and teaches a balance between the will and the ability to surrender.

- Relieves varicose veins.

- Improves circulation to the abdominal organs and legs.

- Strengthens the muscles supporting the joints in the extremities, especially the knees and ankles.

- Opens the hips and chest while strengthening and toning the lower body.

- Stimulates the yoni/female organs, respiratory and cardiovascular systems.

- Grounding.

- Builds self-esteem, courage, and self-worth.

Precautions and Contraindications:

- Those with knee and ankle pain should begin with a modification.

- Inguinal hernia.

- Recent or chronic injury to the legs, hips, back, or shoulders.

Modification

- Stand with your back against the wall.

- Lie on the floor with the soles of your feet pressing against the wall.

Variation: Move your arms into external and internal rotation as you hold the pose.

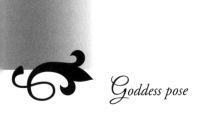

Goddess pose

Warrior/Strength and Wisdom
Sanskrit name: Virabhadrasana

The warrior takes action. The warrior's body moves with force and stands with power, bringing the will into complete focus in order to balance the body. The warrior's heart is made strong by the fire of the spirit. The warrior must know when to take action. In stillness, the body senses the power of its own presence. In the discipline of silence, clarity will come. When observant and patient, the voice knows when to speak. The lengthening of the throat allows the voice to speak with authority. The devoted heart gives meaning to the warrior's purpose. A wise warrior knows that balance of power and will is tempered by wisdom. Does the spirit of the warrior live within you?

Entry and Holding Posture

1. Start with right leg forward first, legs apart, keeping your knee aligned with and over the your ankle.

2. Left foot perpendicular to the right.

3. Crown of head faces up towards the sky, spine strong and erect, arms out, shoulder blades squeezing together, opening the heart, and feet firmly planted on the ground.

4. Drop your tailbone and weight down towards the earth, feeling the strength of your hips and thighs.

5. Pull up on your left kneecap to engage your left thigh; engage your left buttock and press your pelvis forward; feel the surge of power.

6. Lengthen out through both arms, then, looking over your right middle finger, stay focused and breath in and out of your nostrils only, feeling the heat and energy move through your body. See page 226 for photo.

7. Hold up to thirty seconds—about five big belly breaths.

8. Then come into your fire breath: for twenty breaths, breath into your yoni, your female organs, and feel the fire and heat in your belly emerge— your core power .

Repeat on the left side.

Benefits and Systems Being Treated, Challenged, and Healed:

- Strengthens the entire body while improving mental capacity and self-control.

- Builds, shapes, and tones the entire lower body: buttocks, hips, thighs, and ankles.

- Tones and builds the abdominal section.

- Helps to prevent, reduce, and eliminate back pain.

- Strengthens the entire upper body: chest, shoulders, and back.

- Increases the capacity of the respiratory system.

- Stretches the chest, expanding the lung capacity.

Precautions and Contraindications:

- High blood pressure.

- Heart problems.

- Ankle or hip injuries.

Tree Pose/Nourishment
Sanskrit name: Vrikshasana

What nourishes you and provides strength and balance? Are you taking in as much energy and nourishment as you are giving out? Have you hugged a tree today? In this balancing posture, we practice the strength and wisdom of the tree and focus on the third eye to allow our intuition to emerge. The tree is an enlightened being, an avatar of nature. We could not survive without it. The tree's branches reach up toward Father Sky, and the roots reach down to gather nourishment and warmth from Mother Earth. The tree is home to many creatures. The tree provides wood to keep us warm, medicine to heal, fruit to eat, shade, and comfort.

In this pose, your feet are the roots holding you in place. Your legs and spine are the trunk standing firm and sturdy, yet supple. Your arms and fingers are the branches and leaves reaching for sunlight and rain. The heart, like the tree, is an oracle of wisdom. Are you taking in as much energy as you are putting out? Are you able to receive as much as you give?

Entry and Holding Posture

1. Stand with your feet hip-width apart, feet planted firmly into the earth, the crown of your head reaching toward the sky, arms at your sides.

2. Flex your left kneecap to strengthen the left thigh, and lift the right foot to the inside of the left inner thigh.

3. Press your right foot into your left inner thigh.

4. Place your hands in prayer position in front of your heart.

5. Once you find your balance, lift your hands and arms over your head.

6. Breathe in and out through your nostrils only and stare at an object on the ground in front of you to help you balance and focus.

7. If you are having a hard time with balance, place your right foot to the inside of your left ankle.

8. Breathe and hold, then switch legs.

9. Repeat, lifting with the left leg.

Hold up to 15–30 seconds each side—about five big breaths through the nostrils only. Repeat on the other side.

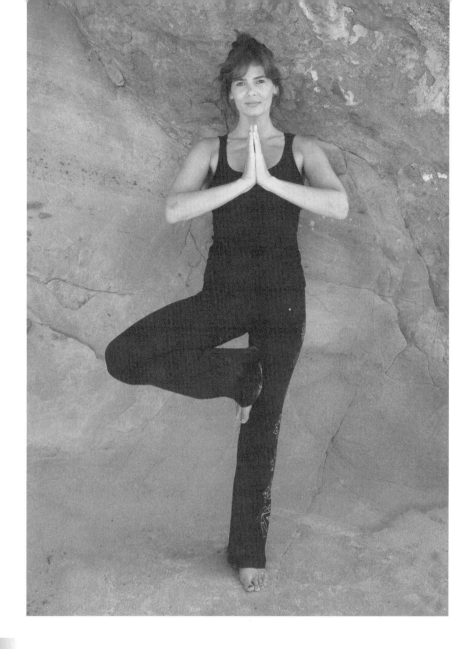

 *Tree pose*

Benefits and Systems Being Treated, Challenged, and Healed:

· Balances the left and right hemispheres of the brain and the male and female energies.

· Strengthens the thighs, buttocks, knees, and ankles.

· Compresses the ovaries and opens the heart.

· Creates inner peace; calms and balances a restless mind. Creates physical balance as well.

· Strengthens legs.

· Increases stamina, improves coordination.

· Great for varicose veins.

· Keeps us in touch with Mother Earth and feeds us vitality.

· Grounds and centers. Taps into our inner wisdom.

Precautions and Contraindications:

· Do not do if you have external hip rotation difficulty.

· Low blood pressure.

· High blood pressure: don't raise arms overhead.

· Heart problems.

Modifications

Use pole or wall for support. Foot may be on the side of ankle or thigh. Hands may remain in prayer position or out to side for balance.

Mountain Pose/Stability
SANSKRIT NAME: TADASANA

Do you know what your morals and values are? Do you know how to stand in your truth? Do you have the stamina, strength, and focus to reach the peak of your mountain, your dreams and visions? The lower body is the base, the foundation. The torso lifts to help the spine climb upward. The heart is an open cave in which to seek silence and solitude. The head is the peak, where answers are discovered. Reach beyond your fears and conquer your dreams. Where do you stand in your life?

Entry and Holding Posture

1. Stand with your feet hip-width apart, heart open, your shoulder blades squeezing together, and your head reaching up toward the sky. Keep your feet, hips, and legs firmly planted into the ground.

2. Lift your arms up to heart level, breathe into your pelvic floor, then lift the breath up into your heart and into your lungs, which extend to the top of your shoulders.

3. Breathe, and feel the power of your breath moving through your body.

4. Proceed to lift your arms overhead, lengthen out through fingertips, and drop your shoulders away from your ears. Breathe in and out through your nostrils only. (See photo, page 100.)

5. Breathe into the sensations, and release what you no longer believe in to lighten the weight on your heart and mind.

Hold up to sixty seconds—about ten big breaths through the nostrils only.

Benefits and Systems Being Treated, Challenged, and Healed:

- Brings the spine into proper alignment.
- Aligns the will of ego with the will of the divine.
- Strengthens core muscles, leading to a healthy digestive tract.
- Expands rib cage, expands lung capacity for better breathing.
- Helps maintain a strong presence in your body and promotes feelings of groundedness.
- Compresses the thymus, strengthening the immune system.
- Releases tension in the neck and shoulders.
- Strengthens thighs, shoulders, and upper back muscles.

Precautions and Contraindications:

- Shoulder injuries.
- Weak lower back.

Body	Element	Exercises & Postures
Physical	Earth	Connecting to the earth, lie on ground or hug a tree, gardening, exercise, weights, hiking, yoga, healthy eating, music, detox, fasting, purification, ceremonies, massage, body work, Reiki, self-healing, mud bath, earth breath Postures: mountain, mother earth, tree, goddess, warrior
Emotional	Water	Dancing, drumming, singing, aromatherapy, bathing in sea salt or natural waters, emotional release work such as hitting a pillow (venting), ocean breath, ha (hara) breath Postures: sphinx, cobra, boat, bow, camel, bridge, wheel
Mental	Air	Holding amethyst crystal, archery, yantra, tratak, journaling, affirmations, breathe lavender in each nostril, labyrinth, nadi breath Postures: eagle, half shoulder stand, plow, locust
Spiritual	Fire	Creating an altar, prayer, ritual, ceremony, offering of gratitude to Spirit and Earth, soul searching, cards and intuition, song or mantra, initiations such as vision quest or sweat lodge, fasting, day of silence and solitude, fire breath Postures: lotus, yoga mudra, posterior stretch, triangle, fish

Areas of Maturity	Core Concepts	Chakras
Grow: Build a foundation of strength and suppleness	Ground and connect	Root: I claim the power of the goddess within me. Sexual: I feel the sensual and sexual energy of the goddess within me.
Love: Give yourself permission to feel	Release and flow	Solar Plexus: I honor, embrace, and embody the goddess within me. Heart: I emanate the spirit of the goddess.
Learn: Learn the discipline of silence and stillness	Balance of intuition and intellect	Throat: I speak the truth of the goddess through me. Third Eye: I recognize the wisdom and magic of the goddess within me.
Evolve: Honor your true nature	Surrender and allow	Crown: I know I am a goddess and recognize my worth; I desire, require, and deserve.

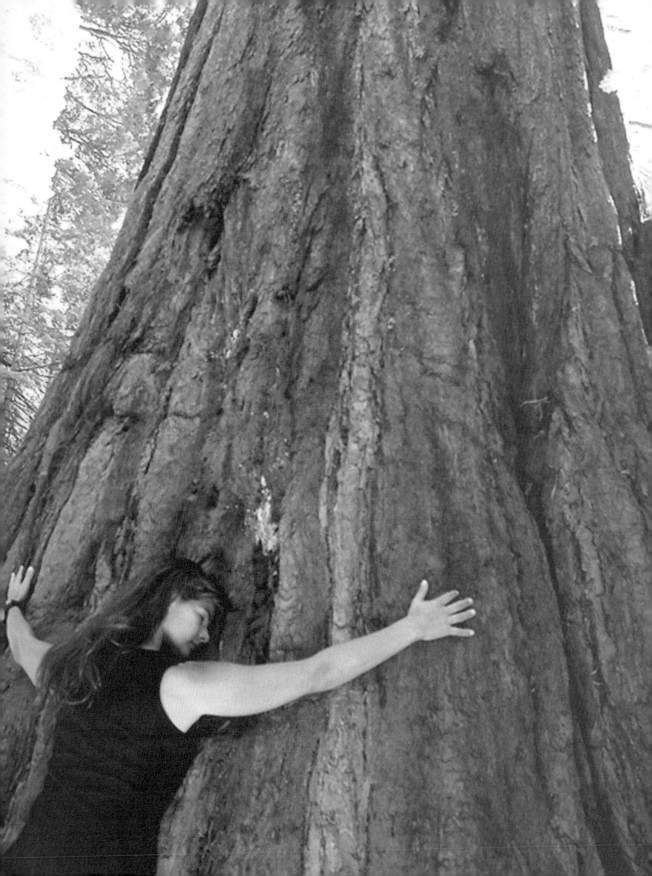

Chapter 6

PUTTING THE FEMALE SPIRIT INTO ACTION

Subconsciously, from birth through adulthood, life's experiences lead you away from your center. Consciously, the 4 Body Fit concept brings you back, showing you how to stop, look, listen, and feel what is going on in all four of your bodies so you can identify and then treat the cause of your discomfort. It will help you understand how to use your intuition, instincts, and senses as pathways to harnessing your body's natural wisdom.

Life is a journey of self-realization, a combination of motion and stillness to create balance in our being. Fitness is more than a workout in a gym or a yoga class; health is more than diet and exercise; and healing is more than facing pain. To be truly fit, we must understand the unique synergy of the physical, mental, emotional, and spiritual bodies to tone the body, awaken the mind, release pent-up emotions, and strengthen our spiritual connection.

In order to do this, we must redefine our concepts of beauty, fitness, and power. In doing so, we create a healthy, balanced model for the twenty-first century. This new definition is simultaneously an internal presence and an external attitude. Beauty is not only a picture-perfect postcard; it is an attitude that is both seen and felt. You create this all-encompassing attitude because you did the work from the inside out.

By removing toxins and stress in our lives, we give our energy permission to be free and cleanse anything within us that does not serve us. This is a discipline and commitment to oneself to create harmony and balance within, even though there is duality around. This discipline allows you to stop, look, listen, and feel. It creates time to retreat, meditate, and pray, moving your attention inward to gain insight and strength as you move forward on your path.

When we take the time to create a space to purify and cleanse ourselves, we regain a sense of our center—our personal energy and power. In this space, we learn a new type of power, the power to let go, to surrender—removing old habits, patterns, beliefs, resentments, and worries, and making room for the positive to come in. This action allows our physical, emotional, and mental energies to rehabilitate our spirit and rebuild our sense of self.

All the tools we have discussed in the earlier chapters have included traditional yoga postures, fitness exercises, breathing exercises, meditation, visualization, music, physiology of disease, nutrition, energetic healing, aromatherapy, and both modern and holistic medicine to create flexibility, strength, focus, suppleness, and full range of motion on all levels of being. The 4 Body Fit concept of driving a car is self-explanatory—we can either *putt-putt* through life as though we have flat tire, or we can move forward and be in the driver's seat to create our own destiny of health, wealth, success, and love.

From reading the chapters, can you see now which of your bodies is overweight or underweight? Which ones you need to work on more to be fully healthy, fit, and empowered? You can now get a feel for what are your personal obstacles, strengths, and weaknesses. Are you present in your body, or are you zoning out—going out of your body? Do you only do what you are best at for fear of failure or discomfort? Do you escape your body or treat your body badly because you do not know how to lose weight, look or feel better? Do you have self-esteem issues that require you to strengthen your core power or do you need to release your creativity or emotions through movement? Being fit, healthy, and whole is so much more than what our media teaches us and gives the body's intelligence credit for. Every day in modern and holistic science, we are continually learning more about all four bodies.

Creating Her-Story

To create a clear image of the female spirit in action, first we must fully define what a twenty-first century goddess looks like, sounds like, and acts like. Let's go back in time—looking at his-tory to create her-story.

The word *goddess* is derived from the word *god*. Goddess is the feminine essence of god. The goddess Durga is also known as Devi to the Indians and Diva to the Italians, from the Latin word *diva*, meaning "goddess," the feminine version of *divus*, meaning "god."

Most of us were taught that God is a man. This is where most religions and spiritual practices have fundamentally failed us. Viewing God as a man takes in only half of the equation of what makes up God, Source, or Spirit. And with something so powerful, it's a shame that we never had the whole thing.

The beauty industry would like us to believe a goddess is only a beautiful woman on a shampoo bottle to sell products or a razor named after a Greek goddess that gives you a close shave for sexy legs. Come on, can we go a little deeper, please? Have you ever asked yourself what a goddess is, or how you feel when you are called a goddess?

In Greek mythology, the goddesses were overridden by the gods. They were forced to be submissive in nature so the gods could grow more powerful. In many religions and countries, many goddess sites of prayer and ceremony were knocked down, with new statues of male gods and the patriarchal systems of religion built upon them, such as churches and other places of prayer.

The goddess dates back to the era between 7000 BC and 3000 BC, a time referred to as Old Europe (Neolithic Europe and Asia Minor), a time when religion had an innate understanding about the wheel of life and its turning—birth, death, and rebirth. They buried their dead in a fetal position, for they knew they were made of the earth and would be born back to the earth, their mother. This is also where the term Mother Earth comes from. Human beings had a deep respect for the earth, which sustained them. The image of the goddess has been found in all cultures in one form or another. She symbolizes the giving and sustaining of life, death, and renewal.

One of the most popular goddess symbols is Venus, the Roman goddess of love (Aphrodite in Greek mythology). A small statuette of a female figure, also known as Venus of Willendorf, was discovered at a Paleolithic site near Willendorf, Austria, and is estimated to have been carved 22,000 to 24,000 years ago. Her arms are reaching up toward the sky, her breasts are full with nutrients and life giving, her belly bountiful and fertile, always giving birth to life. Her vulva (also known as yoni, an Eastern Indian name for the vagina) is the portal to life.

This figure has been seen all over the world. In yoga, it is known as the goddess posture. Women are drawn to this posture because it radiates a peaceful yet fierce presence, a centeredness and connection to Spirit above and earth below—a unity of both forces coming together as one, radiating a power from the inside out.

Ask yourself two questions: What does being feminine mean to me, and what truly is the definition of a goddess to me? Once you can answer this deep within your soul, you can then embrace, embody, and own the power of your feminine essence. You will then know how to put your female spirit into action. Women as a whole cannot move forward until we recognize that our feminine essence is the core of our being—our gift, our worth, and our calling. When we do not recognize this fact, we are only an interpretation of a goddess, a woman who may fall prey to the beauty, medical, and fitness industries that have stripped and depleted us and the earth. Now is the time for women to be warriors of compassion and strength who will lead the battle for the survival and protection of our most important and precious resource: Mother Earth. When we learn to heal ourselves, we also heal the earth. Now is the time to step up to the plate. What are we waiting for?

The time has come to put your female spirit into action and become victorious and courageous, not victimized and compromised.

The female spirit is a magnificent combination of Goddess and Warrior:

- Flexible but firm.

- Graceful yet strong.

- Receptive yet protected.

- Observant yet focused.

- Compassionate and powerful.

- Emotional and intellectual.

- Peaceful yet fierce.

A Goddess Warrior creates her own destiny, rather than allowing her environment to shape her. Her energy comes from a place of centeredness and balance. She is in touch with her intuition and brave enough to follow its guidance.

In order for you to do the necessary work to unleash the goddess within, you're going to have to make a commitment to yourself that you will master the fine art of surrendering and that you will consciously choose to stop, look, and listen to what your deeper inner knowing is telling you anytime your rational mind starts with negative chatter.

To remind yourself of your dedication, copy the following mantra that I wrote onto several index cards and put it in places where you will see it every day—taped to your bathroom mirror, as a bookmark in your daily planner, on the refrigerator, and so on. Say it to yourself many times a day.

Goddess Mantra

I am a twenty-first-century goddess.
I am feminine.
I am sensual.
I am sexual.
I am powerful.
Don't ever mistake my kindness for weakness,
and don't ever take me for granted.

When you have mastered this natural state of being, you will have found your true goddess nature—your goddess to the core. By tapping into your life force, you tap into your own personal energy and power and the connection to the universe within you and surrounding you. Your body becomes a physical vehicle to allow the spirit of God to come through, uniting you with the life force of all the creatures around you, seen and unseen: trees, rocks, mountains, animals, people, angels, spirit guides, planets, stars, water, earth, fire, and air. These are all parts of the universe that will sustain you on your journey. Know that not only is God above and within but also below in Mother Earth, the feminine essence of God.

When you become in tune with the known and the unknown, you will realize that you are never alone. When you open yourself up to the mysteries of the universe, you open your heart to feel your worthiness and open your mind to see your true potential.

If you are unable to go to this place of stillness and silence, then you are unable to manifest and give birth to your dreams and visions. We can no longer sit on the bench.

The time is now to empower ourselves and the next generation. As one woman in our own family, we have the power to change four generations by just shifting our consciousness and no longer accepting the rules that have cuffed our spirits and literally shut us up for thousands of years. That is a lot of power.

Empowerment is a word that means pulling forth what is already within you. The reason for our discomfort in ourselves and world today is that we are in search of empowerment. Where does our power really come from?

The ancient Romans knew that power comes from within. They gave us the word "to educate"—it means to lead out from someone, to bring to the light of day what is already within a person, to coax out the potential for greatness that resides in each person.

The spiral found in the image of the goddess signifies the center from which springs all the streams of feeling and decision making. The goddess knows and teaches others that to be educated means to grow in energy emanating from within each person.

Now is the time for you to go out from here to continue your own empowerment and share it with others. Here you found a place of refreshment and strength, and now you will channel this new energy into all the relationships of your life. Your family and home, your neighborhood, your town or city, even your nation will feel this wave of the future of women in the world. In Goddess we trust! It is time to reclaim, restore, and rejoice in ourselves, to bring balance and unity to each other and to Mother Earth.

Right now, go deep into your belly and find your voice—the rage, anger, disappointment, joy, gratitude, or whatever you are feeling. Allow this voice to be heard, for this is your inner child. She is the intuitive one, the wise one, and the one who will never betray you. She is your power, your voice, and your freedom. She knows how to claim her power. She is the goddess in your core. She is willing to stand naked in the sunlight, claim her power, and declare:

- I did not come here to sleep. I came here to wake up!

- I did not come here to live in pain. I came here to experience pleasure!

- I did not come here to be still. I came here to dance!

- I am not here to watch. I am here to create what I desire, require, and deserve.

- I know and accept that I already am a goddess.

She will constantly remind you to realign with your core through the following three basic guidelines:

First Step:
REDEFINE FITNESS

A goddess knows that being healthy is being fit. She sets goals. She doesn't punish herself by setting unrealistic expectations. She knows that fitness is a journey to take one step at a time, through the body, mind, and spirit.

Body

YOU, the determined woman, have a plan—a cycle of fitness and health that enables you to feel the power of your body.

Mind

YOU, the smart woman, are aware that knowledge is the key to reaching your goals.

Spirit

YOU, the empowered woman, know that power comes from within, not some outside force.

The commitment you make to finding your balance will help find your spiritual fulfillment and lead you on a path to complete wholeness.

Second Step:
REDEFINE BEAUTY

A goddess knows from her core that her internal health gives her the goddess glow that radiates from the inside out. She knows what she does on the inside reflects on the outside. A goddess knows her beauty is not only to be seen but also to be felt, and that her worth is not what she weighs or what she looks like. She is no longer pulled out of her core by the Goddess vs. Barbie syndrome, the inner battle of beauty and power, internal health verses external beauty.

Mirror, mirror, on the wall, you are your mother, after all. Forgive and have gratitude for your mother. She may not have had the same choices you have today. You are both a reflection of love, beauty, grace, anger, and frustration, whether you choose to see it or not. The faster you see it, the faster you will heal. If you are still having problems in your thirties and up, it is time to forgive and move on. You do not have this kind of free time. For those who had a wonderful mother, rejoice in her beauty, grace, and strength. Women as a whole need to heal, stop being a victim, and look at the big picture. Her pain is yours. Her beauty is yours. Her faults are yours. Her gifts are yours.

Third Step:
REDEFINE POWER

A goddess knows her power is not power over, it is power from within. To infuse her attitude with power, she asks herself: *What does being feminine mean to me?*

The goddess no longer thinks that being feminine is being weak. She knows from the core of her being that a goddess pulls higher rank than a princess, diva, or queen. She is not lower than but equal to a king or god, for the goddess is the feminine essence of God. Her power comes from the basic understanding that her true mother is the most powerful goddess of all, Mother Earth. She knows Mother Earth's mystery, magic, wisdom, and wildness is a reflection of the powerful goddess within her, and she knows her birthright is to claim her space.

How to Access, Execute, and Exercise Goddess Power

When you were a little girl, did you get dressed up in your mother's clothes, create imaginary customs, and do role-playing? If so, you were shapeshifting into other forms to become powerful, pretty, outrageous, quirky, and authentic, depending on what the role called for. Many natives use the idea of shapeshifting to travel into other dimensions, worlds that we do not see with common eyes. Shapeshifting is the ability take on strengths and gifts of the seen and unseen worlds to heal and become one with nature and animals, and call upon their powers to help us.

Playing dress-up was so natural—an expression of your creativity, a feeling of freedom to create what you desired by following your imagination. You would embody these characters with heart and soul, and some of us even became these wonderful characters as we grew up.

And that was the question that was always asked: *What do you want to be when you grow up?* I still ask myself this question. I am always transforming myself like a snake shedding its skin. I knew who I was when I was seven, but my projected beliefs took me away from it. I knew I would travel the world, never change my name or get married (I tried it twice, and it didn't work; the divorces lasted longer than the marriages). I knew I would not have children. I knew I would find my partner in my later years. I even had this conversation with my mother, my innate wisdom so clear, pure, and innocent. Eventually, I traveled so far from the truth that it was my near-death experience that took me back to what I knew already at age seven. To this day, I do not have children, I travel the world, I am not married—and I love my life. I do not feel I have missed anything; I have lived a lot in one lifetime already. I know that I am the goddess in her full expression. The little girl in me is the shapeshifter who knows how to play, be creative, and understand the mysteries of the world.

If you have a problem reconnecting to the little girl inside you, ask her to hang out for a day, and she will teach you. Wisdom is not only about age but about truth—being true to yourself is one gift every child has. Did you lose this gift, and if so, when? This is where you were disconnected from your core being, your true authentic self, the God and Goddess within.

In order to find her again, we must first reclaim, restore, and rejoice in who we are as women, and then we can claim our space as goddesses.

Don't be afraid to bend, be flexible, and call upon your gifts to help you through tough times. Men may have a hard time with this since they tend to be so linear. This gift of shapeshifting is truly our power, our expression, and our connection to God. Our flexibility is an outlet for our sensuality to flow when we remember how to dance our own dance.

Before I share some examples on how to use the goddesses in your everyday life, here is a poem written during a boot camp at the Omega Institute in Rhinebeck, New York, by one of the goddess attendees.

The Goddess Journey

by Darina S.

I dreamed of the Goddess
I feared the Goddess
I wanted to be Goddesslike
I ended up living Godlessly

I needed the Goddess
I blamed the Goddess
I've hidden from the Goddess
I learned from the Goddess

I sought the Goddess
I avoided the Goddess
I prayed to the Goddess
I ignored the Goddess

I judged the Goddess
I forgave the Goddess
I imitated the Goddess
I released the Goddess

I admired the Goddess
I envied the Goddess
I felt the Goddess
I resisted the Goddess

I cried with the Goddess
I laughed with the Goddess
I sweated with the Goddess
I danced with the Goddess

I desire to be the Goddess
I require to be the Goddess
I deserve to be the Goddess
I am the Goddess

We are the Goddesses
And so it is.

Kali
EASTERN INDIAN GODDESS OF FEAR

Can't sleep at night? Mulling over the same old stuff over and over again? Kali is here to help you reclaim the lost parts of yourself that you buried away for fear of not being heard, seen, or loved. She asks where you would rather put your energy: faith or fear? Both are unseen, and where you direct your energy is a choice. When we face our fears, we walk through them. Fear is formless. The next time you are scared to face your fears or express your anger or rage, call on Kali. Kali senses what is not in the light of God like a hound dog and brings the fear into the light to heal.

Say you are at a PTA meeting. The school board is discussing the lunches being served, which are full of sugar and carbohydrates because it is cheaper and easier to serve. You know this is unhealthy for your child, yet you have a hard time stepping up to the plate because you do not want to create chaos or confrontation. So you shut your voice and sit with the discomfort and boiling anger churning, which then paralyzes you and ultimately hurts your child.

Remember: if you are unable to protect and provide for yourself, then how in Goddess's name are you going to be able to do this for your child? Think about a lioness who is protecting her cub. Why does something have to be life-threatening before we take action? Why do we wait for a negative force to be right in front of our face and painful before we take action? Guess what, ladies, it's Denial with a capital D. Step up to the plate. A goddess in her power takes action because she is brave enough to follow her intuition, no matter what the consequences. Your intuition will never steer you wrong. Doubt is a dangerous thing that will always cost you in the long run.

Goddess Kali is able to break free from her fear. She cuts through the crap and brings light to any subject. She does not care what others think or do because she knows what the pink elephant in the room is and that it needs to leave. She never defaults to denial. She easily is a Goddess Warrior who can defeat anything that is not pure and light. She brings truth and awareness to any subject so it can heal and shift. She is fierce yet compassionate about her cause and fights to create change. Why is it that a lot of women fear confrontation? Change your perception. Confrontation creates change.

Freya
NORTHERN EUROPEAN GODDESS OF SEXUALITY

Does your relationship need help in the sex department? Call on Freya, the goddess of sensuality, to dance with you between the sheets. Call on her to help you embody the feelings of sexual pleasure and spiritual ecstasy. Allow yourself to open and flow with her in her den, your bedroom. She will show you how to open all your senses—smell, taste, sight, sound, and touch. Your body and your partner's body are awakened by her gifts—aromatic oils, sensual touch and massage, the feeling of a tongue or a feather, enticing music, the sight of evening or morning light, and the taste of exotic foods to help you dance the dance of oneness with your partner. What are you like in bed? You are a mistress, a tigress who requires and deserves ecstatic pleasure back in return.

Artemis
GREEK GODDESS OF SELFHOOD

Feeling burnt out, depleted, and overloaded with chores? Afraid of being alone or not being loved? Are you a worrier or a warrior? Have you lost focus of what you desire and deserve? Call on goddess Artemis, the goddess of self. She represents all aspects of the feminine Goddess Warrior. She is the huntress who shoots her arrows and reaches her goal.

Have you fallen into the role of being codependent or settling because you do not want to be alone? Let Artemis set you free to re-embody your core. Allow her to help you focus on *you*. This is not an act of selfishness but of self-love. Realign yourself with Artemis's target to reach your dreams. She will show you how to be free again. As the huntress of the forest, Artemis knows that love not only comes from humans but from Mother Nature. Take a hike; connect with her through nature, animals, and running free. Artemis stands alone but does not fear her freedom. She knows that her freedom means more to her than anything in the world, even the love of a partner. She is never alone because she has nature and her sisters throughout the world. Artemis asks you: *Self-love or self-pity, which one do you choose?*

Durga/Devi
Eastern Indian Hindu Goddess of Boundaries

Do you know where you begin and where you end? Do you constantly get hurt by others because they are insensitive to your needs? Do you often put others before yourself? Call upon goddess Durga to help you set boundaries. She reminds you that boundaries are not walls. Boundaries are guidelines you share with others to let them know what you will and will not accept. Durga reminds you that people treat you the way you allow them to treat you.

The next time a loved one crosses your boundaries or says or does something inappropriate, call on Durga. She will help you protect your precious space. Her swords and weaponry are her voice. Her body language, her smart-witted mind, and her grace allow her to reflect others' negative energies and demands back at themselves. Her mantra is "Not my shit," which she says to herself internally. Rather than bending to every demand, dart, or arrow, she says, calmly, "How would you like me to respond to that?" She knows how to use energy instead of being used by it.

Next time you have to confront an uncomfortable situation, dodge unhealthy people, or need to stick up for yourself, call on Durga to show you how to set boundaries and set up filters to protect yourself.

Goddess Up!

Many people in the healing business do not know what box to place me in. I am a yoga teacher, energetic healer, medicine woman, therapist, life coach, personal trainer, and psychic. I practice many, yet master none, as they say—but I have mastered how to find Spirit. I use many vehicles to reach divinity, and I do not want to limit myself to only one way to find it. I am open to any experience that will help me grow, learn, love, and evolve—to be my true authentic self. My true medicine is to help people change their perceptions and to experience Spirit in many ways so that they may be truly happy, healthy, and whole—a being who is here to not only be of service to themselves but also to Spirit. I am blessed to do what I do and to help myself and others find their way to their true authentic self.

I have been teaching my Inside-Out Workout and 4 Body Fit system since 1996, right after my near-death experience. I am often asked why I do not work with men.

The answer is quite simple. Generally, men are not willing to work on themselves as much as women, and they have a hard time experiencing fear. Goddesses, going deep is one of our most precious gifts. Just as Eve ate the apple, we are continually searching to better ourselves and our families. We are all natural healers, here to lead. A very powerful native medicine woman told me to have mercy on men because they are born like they are, just as we are born like we are. We must not try to find what is wrong with each other, but what is right.

My biggest fear is that as more and more women come forward and find their Goddess self, they will go back home and judge their men as unworthy. Now that the veil has been lifted, they may feel their partner has failed them, or they may want something new because their partner is not ready to accept change and growth. Before you make any decisions about your future together, let your man read this book so he knows where you are coming from and won't be threatened by your newfound power and beauty. If your partner does not rise to the occasion of finding himself and the relationship feels more like an obstacle than a partnership, then you can make a healthy choice to move on. But remember how long it took you to find self-love in the first place.

By understanding and acknowledging how both energies of the sexes work, we can then respect and trust each other's God-given gifts, thus creating balance within us and surrounding us. Instead of spending so much time trying to change or convince our partners that "this is the way" or "come to my side," we learn how each other's energies work from a very primitive and natural way—how God created us differently.

You must know that the only way to help your loved ones become empowered is by being an example of self-love, not by trying to "fix" anyone. Our job as a goddess and a woman is not to exert power over others but to model the power of self-love. Your challenge is to learn how to be a leader, not a dictator. The world has had enough dictators. And we women can no longer sit on the bench. We need to put our female spirit into action and create change by becoming empowered and by uniting with each other. We need to change the unhealthy perceptions of a woman and her power for the next generation and claim what is legally and humanly ours. When women come together, we can move mountains and create a new story, her-story, and a new way of life.

Aho! Goddess up! Namaste! Blessings!

A GODDESS TO THE CORE

Embrace It, Embody It, Own It

- She knows her beauty is inside and out.
- She is not here to take up space but to claim it.
- She is not only mentally intelligent, she is also emotionally intelligent.
- She is not a victim of life but a co-creator of her life.
- Her sexuality and sensuality are for her to enjoy, not to be used as tools of manipulation.
- She leads by example, not out of fear or control.
- She is feminine but also strong.
- Her attitude is her power.
- Her presence is grace.
- Her intuition and connection to Mother Earth is her core strength.
- The twenty-first-century goddess creates her own destiny. She does not let her surroundings shape her.

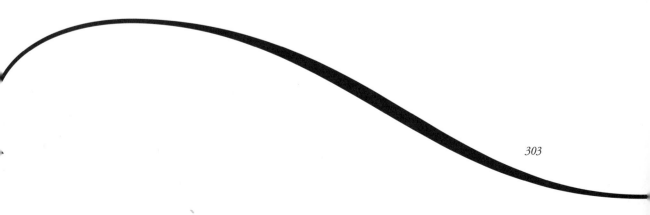

Goddess Secrets
Thirteen Empowering Guidelines

1. You have the right and ability to say *no.*

2. Stop saying *I'm sorry* for something you have no control over.

3. Say yes to pleasure. Rejoice in your sensuality and sexuality.

4. Say yes to power. Being feminine doesn't mean being a pushover.

5. Express, don't suppress. Stop apologizing for being a woman. Emotions are a part of who we are.

6. Draw the line. Take command of your space.

7. Take a stand. Find your voice. Find your courage.

8. Guilt—who needs it? Get off your own case. Guilt is learned, not earned.

9. Stop beating yourself up. Stop setting unrealistic expectations. Who you are is enough.

10. Say goodbye to the "nice girl." Who are you fooling? Be true to yourself. Say what you mean and mean what you say.

11. Face the reality. Superwoman and Supermom are cartoon characters.

12. You are worthy. You are deserving. Learn the rewards of receiving as well as giving.

13. You desire, require, and deserve an abundance of love, money, health, wealth, success, and beauty inside and out.

GODDESS TO THE CORE WORKOUT

Reclaim, Restore, and Rejoice in the Goddess Within

The Six-minute Daily Ritual

1) Spiritual body: Ignite the goddess within.

   STEP 1: Light a candle.

   STEP 2: Set your intention to honor the goddess within.

2) Mental body: Believe in your goddess wisdom.

   STEP 1: Sage yourself to cleanse and release negativity.

   STEP 2: Set your intention for the day.

3) Emotional Body: Embody your goddess power by completing the hara/ha breath (10 each):

   STEP 1: Ha above. Pulling in universal energy.

   STEP 2: Ha below. Pulling in Mother Earth energy.

   STEP 3: Ha middle. Uniting both forces within.

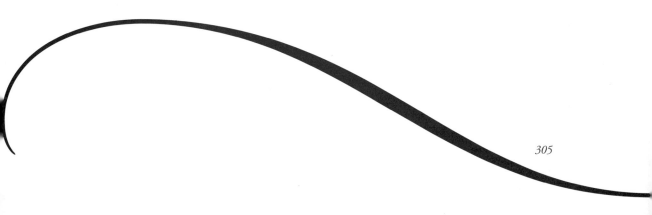

4) Physical body: Own your Goddess Warrior self.

    a) Goddess yoga posture—express out loud (with attitude):

> *I am a twenty-first-century goddess.*
> *I am feminine.*
> *I am sensual.*
> *I am sexual.*
> *I am powerful.*
> *Don't ever mistake my kindness for weakness,*
> *and don't ever take me for granted.*

    b) Goddess and warrior yoga postures, uniting the Goddess and Warrior self.

STEP 1: Start with the goddess posture.

STEP 2: Come into center, hands in prayer position, feet hip-width apart.

STEP 3: Step right leg out to the right side first, claiming your space with the ha breath, then back to center, feet hip-width apart; repeat to the left side.

STEP 4: Next the warrior posture.

STEP 5: Lunge forward on the right leg first, swinging the arms overhead, hands in a fist with the ha breath, then back to center, feet hip-width apart. Repeat on the left side.

STEP 6: Combine both postures in one complete set. Do five sets.

5) Closing:

    a) With hands in prayer position, say the following: (moving hands to the crown of the head) "May I know my truth," (with hands to the third eye) "see my truth," (with hands to the mouth) "speak my truth," (with hands to the heart) "and feel my truth."

    b) Kneel down to Mother Earth and bow, honoring Mother Earth with "Aho!"

    c) Ask, "How can I best be of service to Spirit today?"

REFERENCES

Goddess Books

Apeles, Teena. *Women Warriors: History's Greatest Female Warriors.* Berkeley: Seal Press, 2003.

Bolen, Jean Shinoda, M.D. *Goddesses in Older Women: Archetypes in Women Over Fifty.* New York: Harper Paperbacks, 2002.

De Grandis, Francesca. *Be a Goddess: A Guide to Magical Celtic Spells for Self-Healing, Prosperity and Great Sex.* New York: HarperOne, 1998.

Eldredge, Stasi, and John Eldredge. *Captivating: Unveiling the Mystery of a Woman's Soul.* Nashville: Thomas Nelson, Inc., 2007.

Estés, Clarissa Pinkola, Ph.D. *Women Who Run with the Wolves.* New York: Ballantine Books, 1996.

Gimbutas, Marija. *The Living Goddesses.* Berkeley: University of California Press, 2001.

Muscio, Inga. *Cunt: A Declaration of Independence.* Berkeley: Seal Press, 2002.

Narby, Jeremy. *The Cosmic Serpent.* New York: Penguin Putnam, 1999.

Redmond, Layne. *When the Drummers Were Women: A Spiritual History of Rhythm.* New York: Three Rivers Press, 1997.

Stassinopoulos, Agapi. *Conversations with Goddesses: Revealing the Divine Power within You.* New York: Stewart, Tabori and Chang, 1999.

Tanner, Wilda B. *The Mystical Magical Marvelous World of Dreams*. Tahlequah, OK: Sparrow Hawk Press, 2009.

Walker, Barbara G. *The Women's Encyclopedia of Myths & Secrets*. New York: HarperOne, 1983.

Yoga Books

Radha, Swami Sivananada. *Hatha Yoga (The Hidden Language)*. Kootenay, BC: Timeless Books, 2006.

Yogananda, Paramahansa. *Autobiography of a Yogi*. Los Angeles: Self-Realization Fellowship, 2006.

Healing Books

Borysenko, Joan. *Woman's Book of Life: The Biology, Psychology, and Spirituality of the Feminine Cycle*. New York: Riverhead Books, 1998.

Brennan, Barbara. *Hands of Light: A Guide to Healing Through the Human Energy Field*. New York: Bantam, 1988.

———. *Light Emerging: The Journey of Personal Healing*. New York: Bantam, 1993.

Frost, Peter J. *Toxic Emotions at Work*. Boston: Harvard Business School Press, 2007.

Hay, Louise L. *You Can Heal Your Life*. Carlsbad, CA: Hay House, Inc., 1984.

———. *Heal Your Body A–Z*. Carlsbad, CA: Hay House, Inc., 2001.

Judith, Anodea. *Wheels of Life: A User's Guide to the Chakra System*. St. Paul: Llewellyn Publications, 1999.

Spalding, Baird. *Life and Teaching of the Masters of the Far East*. Camarillo, CA: DeVorss & Company, 1978.

Native Books

Andrews, Ted. *Animal-Speak*. St. Paul, MN: Llewellyn Publications, 1996.

McGaa, Ed (Eagle Man). *Mother Earth Spirituality: Native American Paths to Healing Ourselves and Our World*. New York: HarperCollins Publishers, 1990.

Sams, Jamie, and David Carson. *Medicine Cards* (deck of cards and book). New York: St. Martin's Press, 1988.

Aromatherapy

Higley, Connie, and Alan Higley. *Reference Guide for Essential Oils*. Abundant Health, 2008.

Others

Arewa, Caroline Shola. *Opening to Spirit*. London: Thorsons, 1999.

Davis, Wade. *The Serpent and the Rainbow*. New York: Simon & Schuster, 1997.

Eldredge, John. *Wild at Heart: Discovery of a Man's Soul*. Nashville: Thomas Nelson Inc., 2006

Farrell, Warren. *Why Men Are the Way They Are*. New York: Berkley Publishing, 1988.

Hanley, Kate. *The Anywhere, Anytime Chill Guide*. Guilford, CT: Globe Pequot Press, 2008.

Marashinsky, Amy Sophia. *The Goddess Oracle Deck of Cards*. U.S. Games Systems, 2006.

Melody. *Love Is in the Earth: A Kaleidoscope of Crystals*. Wheat Ridge, CO: Earth Love Publishing House, 1995.

Sui, Choa Kok. *Advanced Pranic Healing*. Sterling Publishers, India: 2000.

Williamson, Marianne. *A Woman's Worth*. New York: Random House Publishing Group, 1994.

———. *A Return to Love: Reflections on the Principles of "A Course in Miracles."* New York: Harper, 1996.

INDEX

245–246, 249, 254, 256, 260, 276, 285

inside-out workout, 61, 133, 193, 254, 301

intelligence, xiv, xvii, 12–14, 35–36, 48–49, 52–54, 60, 81, 104, 108, 110–113, 117, 126–128, 132, 135, 142–143, 163–164, 166–167, 171, 174–175, 191, 193, 195, 203, 227–228, 238, 241, 244–246, 254, 256, 290

intuition, vi, xiv–xv, xvii, 4, 13, 18, 25, 34, 36, 41, 44–46, 49, 52–55, 57, 59–60, 64–66, 71–72, 74, 78, 81, 84–86, 89, 91, 105, 107, 111, 113, 116, 119, 125–130, 132, 135–138, 143, 147, 163, 166, 172, 174, 182–183, 186, 198, 203, 222, 228, 231, 247, 254, 265, 269, 282, 286, 289, 293, 299, 303

itty-bitty shitty committee, 114, 121–124

journaling, 144–145, 286

Kali, 36, 138, 299

karma, 30, 78, 113, 121, 183, 240

Kenzo, Awa (Zen archery master), 146

Ki, xiv, 32, 258

Kripalu Center for Yoga & Health, xvi

kundalini, xiv, 4, 25, 27, 45, 75, 115, 138

labyrinth, 72, 115, 134–135, 269, 271, 286

lavender essential oil, 140–142

left brain, 113

life force, 4, 7, 27, 48–49, 51–53, 55, 60, 62, 73, 102, 139, 142, 162, 172, 182, 196, 198, 202–203, 230, 233, 244, 246, 256, 264, 293

Lilith, 23–25, 27

main systems of the body, 238

mantras, vii, xiii, 63, 74–75, 78–79, 107, 128, 178–179, 277, 286, 293, 301
   goddess, 178, 277, 293

masculine, xvi, 25, 27, 33–34, 40–43, 111, 113

mask, 116–119, 196, 243

massage, xiii, 43, 49, 85, 139–140, 157, 193–195, 235, 258–259, 286, 300

maze, 72, 114–115, 134

meditation, xiii, xv–xvi, 17, 54, 71, 73–74, 78–79, 84, 89, 128, 183, 188, 290

menopause, 4, 56, 99, 157, 252

midlife crisis, 56

Mother Earth
   exercises to connect to, 264

muscle memory, 239

music, 48, 83, 114, 130, 145, 186, 257, 260–261, 286, 290, 300

nadi breath, 147, 286